BSAVA
Pocketbook for Vets

Editor:
Sheldon Middleton
MA VetMB MRCVS

BSAVA
BRITISH SMALL ANIMAL
VETERINARY ASSOCIATION

Published by:
British Small Animal Veterinary Association
Woodrow House, 1 Telford Way, Waterwells Business Park,
Quedgeley, Gloucester GL2 2AB

A Company Limited by Guarantee in England.
Registered Company No. 2837793.
Registered as a Charity.

Other BSAVA Member benefits

For further information on any of the below benefits of membership email administration@bsava.com, or call 01452 726700.

■ Congress discount

The BSAVA is committed to making its Congress a real benefit for members when it comes to cost. Members also receive their registration packs earlier than anyone else to make sure they get preferential access to masterclasses and social tickets.

■ Congress Podcasts

An archive of lectures covering a range of small animal topics from the last few years of Congress. BSAVA members can listen online or download to their iPod/MP3 player.

■ CPD discount

High standards and low costs are the BSAVA's key aims when delivering CPD throughout the UK. We send the annual brochure to members in advance of the general release so you won't miss out on the course you want. Prices are approximately 30% lower for members.

■ Publications discount

More and more new titles and editions are released every year. Members get these invaluable and popular additions to their veterinary library at great discounts, making it one of the key benefits of membership.

■ *BSAVA Small Animal Formulary*

This indispensable pocket guide is now in its 7th edition. Every vet member receives a free copy when they join and a free copy of each new edition. Also available as online searchable version and as a Smartphone App for vet members (login required for both).

■ *Journal of Small Animal Practice*

Members' free subscription to *Journal of Small Animal Practice* (JSAP) gives them invaluable access to all the latest research and scientific advancements within the profession. Student members only have online access. Members are also entitled to free online access to *The European Journal of Companion Animal Practice* via the FECAVA website.

■ companion

This publication for all BSAVA members provides practical content which relates to your needs in practice. **companion** delivers accessible, instructive CPD features, articles on the issues that are facing the profession and of course, general Association news.

■ Health and Safety resource

A comprehensive resource containing downloadable templates and guidelines providing members with a structure that can be used to create individual health and safety documents, processes and policies for their particular circumstances.

➤

■ Medicines information: client leaflets

A series of downloadable information leaflets which can be used to advise your clients about the safe use of the drugs that you prescribe and dispense for the patients under their care.

■ Regional CPD meetings

BSAVA has 12 regions covering the UK, run by committed volunteers. Members can access regional CPD at reduced prices, meet other local professionals and even get involved in choosing the subjects covered in the programme.

■ Free room hire

Ideal for interviews or staff training days, members can benefit from free room hire during office hours (9am – 5pm), Monday to Friday at BSAVA Headquarters with meeting solutions for up to 40 delegates. Catering can be supplied as an extra cost and should you require the meeting facilities outside office hours, this can be organised at a supplementary cost. For full details and to discuss your requirements, please contact Carole Haile, telephone: 01452 726717, email: c.haile@bsava.com.

■ Professional representation

At a time when the profession is subject to so much change and scrutiny, it has never been more important to make sure your views are represented at the highest level. Every time the Association takes part in a consultation, our members' views are canvassed and considered in the BSAVA's response.

Loyalty Benefits

■ Bonus book

Members will qualify for a bonus book each year that they renew their membership. Bonus books will be available to collect at Congress each year or will be posted soon after if you are unable to attend Congress.

■ VetMed Resource

Access to an online database of veterinary science featuring over 1.4 million bibliographic records across the veterinary sciences plus reseach articles and full text articles dedicated to companion animals. The ideal support for veterinary continuing education. Available to all paying members with two continuous years of membership.

■ Congress Podcast DVD

All paying members with three consecutive years of membership will receive a DVD containing all podcasts from the previous year's Congress.

Contents

➤

Foreword

I am honoured to have been asked to write the Foreword for the first edition of the *BSAVA Pocketbook for Vets*.

There is now a wealth of information available for the vet but, in my experience as a practitioner, there is still a need for immediately concise and accurate information. This pocketbook fills that need. In the digital era there are a number of ways of obtaining information but it will be some time before such methods will replace the pocketbook.

This book includes a wide range of information – from algorithms on pyoderma to biological data on skunks and dosages for reptiles – and yet it is small enough so that it need never leave your side.

The team behind this publication has produced an exceptional guide that allows very rapid access to information and saves that most important commodity for a new graduate and the experienced vet – time. I wish it had been available when I first qualified, and even after all my time in practice I know it will be in my scrubs pocket for immediate reference.

This pocketbook combined with the *BSAVA Small Animal Formulary*, *BSAVA Guide to Procedures in Small Animal Practice* and *BSAVA/VPIS Guide to Common Canine and Feline Poisons* are sufficient reasons alone to join BSAVA as a new graduate.

Mark R. Johnston
BVetMed MRCVS

BSAVA President 2012–13

Preface

The *BSAVA Pocketbook for Vets* is a new initiative from the Membership Development Committee of the BSAVA in response to members' feedback. It is intended to be a 'quick glance' reference that can be carried in a scrub top pocket for ease of use when consulting or during ward rounds. It is not intended to replace the *Formulary* or other BSAVA Manuals but rather to complement them. It is almost impossible to create a reference that will be equally applicable in all clinical settings and so there are notes pages throughout to allow the book to be personalized.

I would like to thank the editorial team and the Publications Committee at BSAVA for their help and guidance when preparing this pocketbook. I would also like to thank and acknowledge the huge number of BSAVA authors whose work I have harvested from other Manuals and articles for inclusion here. Without these people this book could not exist.

Finally, as this is the first edition and a new venture, I would welcome suggestions for inclusion (and teething problems for exclusion!) in future editions. Please contact me at **vetpocketbook@bsava.com**.

Sheldon Middleton
MA VetMB MRCVS

Bedford
May 2012

A few notes on using this book

- Under the drug listings, only doses are mentioned; the more detailed information on contraindications, interactions, etc., can be found in the *BSAVA Small Animal Formulary*. This is to enable the information to be found quickly and to keep the bulk of the book down.

- Selected drugs are listed by generic name. (An index of trade names is provided at the back of the book.)
  - The rINN generic name is used.
  - The list of trade names is not necessarily comprehensive, and the mention or exclusion of any particular commercial product is not a recommendation or otherwise as to its value. Any omission of a product that is authorized for a particular small animal indication is purely accidental.
  - Products that are not authorized for veterinary use by the Veterinary Medicines Directorate are marked with an asterisk. Note that an indication that a product is authorized does not necessarily mean that it is authorized for all species and indications listed in the monograph; users should check individual data sheets.

- Drug doses are based on those recommended by the manufacturers in their data sheets and package inserts, **or** are based on those given in published articles or textbooks, **or** are based on clinical experience. These recommendations should be used only as guidelines and should not be considered appropriate for every case. Clinical judgement must take precedence. Where possible, doses have been given for individual species; however, sometimes generalizations are used. 'Small mammals' includes ferrets, lagomorphs and rodents. 'Birds' includes psittacines, raptors, pigeons and others. 'Reptiles' includes chelonians, lizards and snakes. Except where indicated, all doses given for ectothermic animals (reptiles) assume that the animal is kept within its Preferred Optimum Temperature Zone (POTZ). Animals that are maintained at different temperatures may have different rates of metabolism and therefore the dose (and especially the frequency) that is required may require alteration.

- A veterinary surgeon should always refer to other source material if they are not familiar with the drugs mentioned in this guide.
- The tables of tablet sizes for various weights of animal are taken from the datasheets of certain authorized brands of the drug and are identified as such. Where several brands of the same drug use different sized tablets and have each produced a different table, only one has been included. If this is not the brand used in your clinic, I would encourage you to use the blank pages to personalize your guide.
- Likewise, an algorithm for suggested course of investigation of a certain disease should not be considered in isolation but should be used in context with the relevant Manual or other source material.
- All sources used in this guide are referenced by a superscript number which refers to a bibliography at the back of the book.

Acepromazine [16] (ACP)
(ACP) POM-V

Formulations:
- Injectable: 2 mg/ml solution.
- Oral: 10 mg, 25 mg tablets.

DOSES

Dogs (not Boxers), Cats: 0.01–0.02 mg/kg slowly i.v.;
0.01–0.05 mg/kg i.m., s.c.; 1–3 mg/kg p.o.
- Boxers: 0.005–0.01 mg/kg i.m. or avoid.

Small mammals:
- Ferrets: 0.2–0.5 mg/kg i.m., s.c., p.o.
- Rabbits: 0.1–1.0 mg/kg i.m., s.c.
- Guinea pigs: 2.5–5 mg/kg i.m., s.c., p.o.
- Hamsters: 5 mg/kg i.m., s.c., p.o.
- Gerbils: 3 mg/kg i.m., s.c., p.o.
- Rats: 2.5 mg/kg i.m., s.c., p.o.
- Mice: 1–5 mg/kg i.m., s.c., p.o.

Birds: Not recommended.

Reptiles: 0.1–0.5 mg/kg i.m.

Activated charcoal *see* Charcoal

Amlodipine [16]
(Amlodipine*, Istin*) POM

Formulations: Oral: 5 mg, 10 mg tablets.

DOSES

Dogs: Initial dose 0.05–0.1 mg/kg p.o. q12–24h. The dose may be titrated upwards weekly as required, up to 0.4 mg/kg, monitoring blood pressure regularly.

Cats: 0.625–1.25 mg/cat p.o. q24h. The dose may be increased slowly or the frequency increased to q12h if necessary. Blood pressure monitoring is essential.

Amoxicillin [16] (Amoxycillin)

(Amoxinsol, Amoxival, Amoxycare, Amoxypen, Bimoxyl, Clamoxyl, Duphamox, Vetremox) POM-V

Formulations:

- Injectable: 150 mg/ml suspension.
- Oral: 40 mg, 200 mg, 250 mg tablets; suspension which when reconstituted provides 50 mg/ml.

DOSES

Dogs, Cats:

- Parenteral: 7 mg/kg i.m. q24h; 15 mg/kg i.m. q48h for depot preparations.
- Oral: 10 mg/kg p.o. q8–12h.
- (Doses of 16–33 mg/kg i.v. q8h are used in humans to treat serious infections.) Dose chosen will depend on site of infection, causal organism and severity of the disease.

Clamoxyl Palatable Tablets (from datasheet)			
Species	Dose rate	No. of tablets per dose, twice daily	
		40 mg	*200 mg*
Dogs	4–10 mg/kg twice daily	1–2 per 10 kg bodyweight	½–1 per 20 kg bodyweight
Cats		½–1	

NOTES

Small mammals:
- Ferrets: 10–30 mg/kg s.c., p.o. q12h.
- Rats, Mice: 100–150 mg/kg i.m., s.c. q12h.

Birds: 150–175 mg/kg i.m., s.c. q8–12h (q24h for long-acting preparations)
- Parrots, Raptors: 150–175 mg/kg p.o. q12h.
- Pigeons: 1–1.5 g/l drinking water (Vetremox Pigeon) q24h for 3–5 days or 100–200 mg/kg p.o. q6–8h.
- Waterfowl: 1 g/l drinking water (Amoxinsol soluble powder) alternate days for 3–5 days, 300–500 mg/kg soft food for 3–5 days.
- Passerines: 1.5 g/l drinking water (Vetremox Pigeon).

Reptiles: 5–10 mg/kg i.m., p.o. q12–24h (most species)
- Chelonians: 5–50 mg/kg i.m., p.o. q12h.

Amoxicillin/Clavulanate [16] (Amoxycillin/Clavulanic acid)

(Clavaseptin, Clavoral, Clavucil, Clavudale, Nisamox, Noroclav, Synulox, Augmentin*) POM-V, POM

Formulations:
- Injectable: 175 mg/ml suspension (140 mg amoxicillin, 35 mg clavulanate); 600 mg powder (500 mg amoxicillin, 100 mg clavulanate); 1.2 g powder (1 g amoxicillin, 200 mg clavulanate) for reconstitution (Augmentin).
- Oral: 50 mg, 250 mg, 500 mg tablets each containing amoxicillin and clavulanate in a ratio of 4:1. Palatable drops which when reconstituted with water provide 40 mg amoxicillin and 10 mg clavulanic acid per ml.

DOSES

Dogs, Cats:

- Parenteral: 8.75 mg/kg (combined) i.v. q8h, i.m., s.c. q24h.
- Oral: 12.5–25 mg/kg (combined) p.o. q8–12h.
- (Doses up to 25 mg/kg i.v. q8h are used to treat serious infections in humans.)

➥

Clavucil, Synulox (from datasheets)			
Dose rate	Patient bodyweight (kg)	No. of tablets per dose, twice daily	
		50 mg	*250 mg*
Dogs and cats			
12.5 mg/kg q12h	1–2	½	
	3–5	1	
	6–9	2	
	10–13	3	
	14–18	4	
	19–25		1
	26–35		1½
	36–49		2
	50		3

Small mammals:

- Ferrets: 12.5–20 mg/kg i.m., s.c. q12h.
- Rats, Mice: 100 mg/kg q12h.

Birds: 125–150 mg/kg p.o., i.v. q12h; 125–150 mg/kg i.m. q24h.

NOTES

Ampicillin [16]

(Amfipen, Ampicare, Duphacillin) POM-V

Formulations:

- Injectable: Ampicillin sodium 250 mg, 500 mg powders for reconstitution (human licensed product only); 150 mg/ml suspension, 100 mg/ml long-acting preparation.
- Oral: 500 mg tablets; 250 mg capsule.

DOSES

Dogs:

- Routine infections: 10–20 mg/kg i.v., i.m., s.c., p.o. q6–8h.
- CNS or serious bacterial infections: up to 40 mg/kg i.v. q6h has been recommended.

Cats: 10–20 mg/kg i.v., i.m., s.c., p.o. q6–8h.

Small mammals:

- Ferrets: 5–30 mg/kg i.m., s.c. q12h.
- Rabbits, Chinchillas, Guinea pigs, Hamsters: *do not use*
- Gerbils: 20–100 mg/kg s.c. q8h; 6–30 mg/kg p.o. q8h.
- Rats, Mice: 25 mg/kg i.m., s.c. q12h; 50–200 mg/kg p.o. q12h.

Birds: 50–100 mg/kg i.v., i.m. q8–12h; 150–200 mg/kg p.o. q8–12h; 1–2 g/l drinking water; 2–3 g/kg soft feed.

Reptiles: 20 mg/kg s.c., i.m. q24h at 26°C.

Anaphylaxis – emergency treatment [3]
Identification

Anaphylaxis is an acute severe allergic reaction characterized by venous and arteriolar dilation and increased capillary permeability, which result in decreased venous return to the heart, hypotension and hypovolaemia. Signs of hypovolaemic shock may be associated with:

- Angioedema: this commonly results in facial swelling and swelling of the distal limbs but can include pharyngeal and laryngeal swelling
- Bronchospasm
- Pruritus
- Urticaria: raised red skin wheals or hives
- Vomiting.

➤

Procedure

1. Establish and maintain an airway: intubate if necessary.
2. Check the animal's breathing: administer 100% oxygen via a non-rebreathing mask if dyspnoea is present without airway obstruction.
3. Place a large intravenous catheter.
4. Adrenaline (0.02 mg/kg slowly i.v or into the trachea via an endotracheal tube if intravenous access is not available) should be given in life-threatening cases. Continuous monitoring of cardiovascular status for adrenaline-induced arrhythmias and hypertension and response to therapy is required.
5. Treat hypovolaemic shock with intravenous fluid therapy. Intravenous fluid therapy should be tapered to the individual and determined by continuous cardiovascular and respiratory assessment of the patient to achieve and maintain cardiovascular stability. As a guide, shock boluses of crystalloids (90 ml/kg/h for a dog and 60 ml/kg/h for a cat) may be required initially. Supplemental boluses of colloids (10 ml/kg/h for a dog and 6 ml/kg/h for a cat) may also be required during initial stabilization. Maintenance therapy may require a combination of crystalloids and colloids due to ongoing fluid losses into the interstitium.
6. In animals with hypotension confirmed by blood pressure measurement, which has not responded to steps 4 and 5, vasopressors such as dobutamine (5–15 µg/kg/min) or dopamine (3–10 µg/kg/min) may be required. Treatment with these drugs requires frequent or continuous blood pressure measurement.
7. In animals with bronchospasm and life-threatening angioedema, including laryngeal oedema, dexamethasone (1–2 mg/kg i.v.) and diphenhydramine (0.5–1 mg/kg slow i.v. or i.m.) may be useful adjunctive treatments.
8. Identification and avoidance of the causative factor is important for long-term management.

Apomorphine [16]
(APO-go*) POM

Formulations: Injectable: 10 mg/ml solution in 2 ml or 5 ml ampoules; 5 mg/ml, 10 mg/ml solutions in 10 ml pre-filled syringes.

DOSES

Dogs: 20–40 μg (micrograms)/kg i.v., 40–100 μg/kg s.c., i.m. (i.v. route most effective, i.m. least effective).

Cats: Not recommended; xylazine is a potent emetic in cats and at least as safe.

Small mammals: Do not use.

ASA scale [4]

ASA scale	Physical description	Veterinary patient examples
1	Normal patient with no disease	Healthy patient for ovariohysterectomy or castration
2	Patient with mild systemic disease that does not limit normal function	Controlled diabetes mellitus, mild cardiac valve insufficiency
3	Patient with severe systemic disease that limits normal function	Uncontrolled diabetes mellitus, symptomatic heart disease
4	Patient with severe systemic disease that is a constant threat to life	Sepsis, organ failure, heart failure
5	Patient that is moribund and not expected to live 24 hours without surgery	Shock, multiple-organ failure, severe trauma
E	Describes patient as an emergency	Gastric dilatation–volvulus, respiratory disease

American Society of Anesthesiologists scale of physical status.

Atipamezole [16]

(Alzane, Antisedan, Atipam, Revertor, Sedastop) POM-V

Formulations: Injectable: 5 mg/ml solution.

DOSES

Dogs: Five times the previous medetomidine or dexmedetomidine dose i.m. (i.e. equal volume of solution to medetomidine or dexmedetomidine). When medetomidine or dexmedetomidine has been administered at least an hour before, dose of atipamezole can be reduced by half (i.e. half the volume of medetomidine or dexmedetomidine) and repeated if recovery is slow.

Cats: Two and a half times the previous medetomidine or dexmedetomidine dose i.m. (i.e. half the volume of medetomidine or dexmedetomidine given).

Small mammals: Five times the previous medetomidine dose s.c., i.m., i.v.; 0.5–1 mg/kg i.m., i.p., s.c.

Birds: 0.065–0.25 mg/kg i.m.

Reptiles: Five times the previous medetomidine or dexmedetomidine dose i.m., i.v.

NOTES

NOTES

NOTES

NOTES

NOTES

Benazepril [16]

(Banacep, Benazacare, Bexepril, Fortekor, Nelio, Prilben) POM-V

Formulations: Oral: 2.5 mg, 5 mg, 20 mg tablets.

DOSES

Dogs: Heart failure: 0.25–0.5 mg/kg p.o. q24h.

Cats: Chronic renal insufficiency: 0.5–1.0 mg/kg p.o. q24h.

Fortekor (from datasheet)							
Dose rate	Patient bodyweight (kg)	No. of tablets required					
		2.5 mg		5 mg		20 mg	
		SD	DD	SD	DD	SD	DD
Dogs							
0.25–0.5 mg/kg q24h	2.5–<5	0.5	1				
	5–10	1	2	0.5	1		
	11–20			1	2		
	21–40					0.5	1
	41–80					1	2
Cats							
0.5–1.0 mg/kg q24h	2.5–5	1					
	>5–10	2					

SD = Standard dose; DD = Double dose

Rabbits: Starting dose 0.05 mg/kg p.o. q24h. Dose may be increased to a maximum of 0.1 mg/kg.

Blood pressure *see* **Hypertension**

Body condition score [12]

The Nestlé Purina Body Condition Systems for Dogs and Cats are illustrated on the following pages. Other body condition scoring systems exist, such as the Waltham® S.H.A.P.E.™ Guide for Dogs and the Waltham® S.H.A.P.E.™ Guide for Cats.

■ Nestlé PURINA
Body Condition System for dogs

TOO THIN

1 Ribs, lumbar vertebrae, pelvic bones and all bony prominences evident from a distance. No discernible body fat. Obvious loss of muscle mass.

2 Ribs, lumbar vertebrae and pelvic bones easily visible. No palpable fat. Some evidence of other bony prominence. Minimal loss of muscle mass.

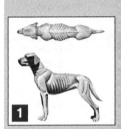

3 Ribs easily palpated and may be visible with no palpable fat. Tops of lumbar vertebrae visible. Pelvic bones becoming prominent. Obvious waist and abdominal tuck.

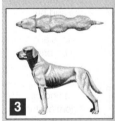

IDEAL

4 **Ribs easily palpable, with minimal fat covering. Waist easily noted, viewed from above. Abdominal tuck evident.**

5 **Ribs palpable without excess fat covering. Waist observed behind ribs when viewed from above. Abdomen tucked up when viewed from side.**

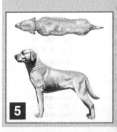

TOO HEAVY

6 Ribs palpable with slight excess fat covering. Waist is discernible viewed from above but is not prominent. Abdominal tuck apparent.

7 Ribs palpable with difficulty; heavy fat cover. Noticeable fat deposits over lumbar area and base of tail. Waist absent or barely visible. Abdominal tuck may be present.

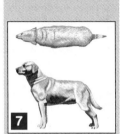

8 Ribs not palpable under very heavy fat cover, or palpable only with significant pressure. Heavy fat deposits over lumbar area and base of tail. Waist absent. No abdominal tuck. Obvious abdominal distention may be present.

9 Massive fat deposits over thorax, spine and base of tail. Waist and abdominal tuck absent. Fat deposits on neck and limbs. Obvious abdominal distention.

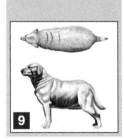

9-point body condition scale for dogs. (© Nestlé Purina PetCare and reproduced with their permission.)

THE BODY CONDITION SYSTEM was developed at the Nestlé Purina Pet Care Center and has been validated as documented in the following publications:

Mawby D, Bartges JW, Moyers T, *et. al.* **Comparison of body fat estimates by dual-energy x-ray absorptiometry and deuterium oxide dilution in client owned dogs.** Compendium 2001; 23 (9A): 70

Laflamme DP. **Development and Validation of a Body Condition Score System for Dogs.** Canine Practice July/August 1997; 22: 10–15

Kealy, *et. al.* **Effects of Diet Restriction on Life Span and Age-Related Changes in Dogs.** JAVMA 2002; 220: 1315–1320

▦ Nestlé PURINA
Body Condition System for cats

TOO THIN

1 Ribs visible on shorthaired cats; no palpable fat; severe abdominal tuck; lumbar vertebrae and wings of ilia easily palpated.

2 Ribs easily visible on shorthaired cats; lumbar vertebrae obvious with minimal muscle mass; pronounced abdominal tuck; no palpable fat.

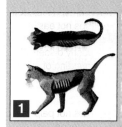

3 Ribs easily palpable with minimal fat covering; lumbar vertebrae obvious; obvious waist behind ribs; minimal abdominal fat.

4 Ribs palpable with minimal fat covering; noticeable waist behind ribs; slight abdominal tuck; abdominal fat pad absent.

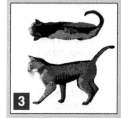

IDEAL

5 **Well-proportioned; observe waist behind ribs; ribs palpable with slight fat covering; abdominal fat pad minimal.**

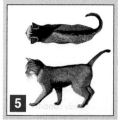

TOO HEAVY

6 Ribs palpable with slight excess fat covering; waist and abdominal fat pad distinguishable but not obvious; abdominal tuck absent.

7 Ribs not easily palpated with moderate fat covering; waist poorly discernible; obvious rounding of abdomen; moderate abdominal fat pad.

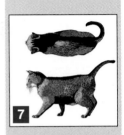

8 Ribs not palpable with excess fat covering; waist absent; obvious rounding of abdomen with prominent abdominal fat pad; fat deposits present over lumbar area.

9 Ribs not palpable under heavy fat cover; heavy fat deposits over lumbar area, face and limbs; distention of abdomen with no waist; extensive abdominal fat deposits.

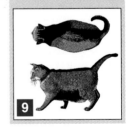

9-point body condition scale for cats. (© Nestlé Purina PetCare and reproduced with their permission.)

Bodyweight (BW) to body surface area (BSA) conversion tables[16]

Dogs

BW (kg)	BSA (m^2)	BW (kg)	BSA (m^2)	BW (kg)	BSA (m^2)
0.5	0.06	11	0.49	24	0.83
1	0.1	12	0.52	26	0.88
2	0.15	13	0.55	28	0.92
3	0.2	14	0.58	30	0.96
4	0.25	15	0.6	35	1.07
5	0.29	16	0.63	40	1.17
6	0.33	17	0.66	45	1.26
7	0.36	18	0.69	50	1.36
8	0.4	19	0.71	55	1.46
9	0.43	20	0.74	60	1.55
10	0.46	22	0.78		

Cats

BW (kg)	BSA (m^2)	BW (kg)	BSA (m^2)	BW (kg)	BSA (m^2)
0.5	0.06	2.5	0.184	4.5	0.273
1	0.1	3	0.208	5	0.292
1.5	0.134	3.5	0.231	5.5	0.316
2	0.163	4	0.252	6	0.33

NOTES

Bromhexine [16]
(Bisolvon) POM-V

Formulations:
- Injectable: 3 mg/ml solution.
- Oral: 10 mg/g powder.

DOSES

Dogs: 3–15 mg/dog i.m. q12h; 2–2.5 mg/kg p.o. q12h.

Cats: 3 mg/cat i.m. q24h; 1 mg/kg p.o. q24h.

Bisolvon (from datasheet)				
Dose of bromhexine HCl	Patient bodyweight (kg)	Dose of Bisolvon Powder (g)	No. of blue (0.5 g) scoops	Frequency and duration
Dogs				
2 mg/kg	5	0.5	1	Twice daily for 5 days
	15	1.5	3	
Cats				
1 mg/kg	5	0.5	1	Once daily for 7 days

Small mammals: 0.3 mg/animal p.o. q24h.

Birds: 1.5 mg/kg i.m., p.o. q12–24h.

Reptiles: 0.1–0.2 mg/kg q24h.

Buprenorphine [16]
(Buprecare, Buprenodale, Vetergesic) POM-V CD Schedule 3

Formulations: Injectable: 0.3 mg/ml solution; available in 1 ml vials that do not contain a preservative, or in 10 ml multidose bottle that contains chlorocresol as preservative.

DOSES

Dogs: 0.02 mg/kg i.v., i.m., s.c. q6h.

Cats: Doses as for dogs. Also well tolerated and effective when given sublingually. ➡

Small mammals:
- Ferrets: 0.01–0.10 mg/kg s.c., i.m., i.v. q8–12h.
- Rabbits: 0.01–0.05 mg/kg s.c., i.m., i.v. q6–12h (doses <0.03 mg/kg have very limited analgesic effects but still have some sedative effects).
- Guinea pigs, Gerbils, Hamsters, Rats: 0.01–0.05 mg/kg i.m., s.c. q6–12h.
- Mice: 0.05–0.1 mg/kg i.m., s.c. q6–12h.

Birds: 0.01–0.05 mg/kg i.v., i.m q8–12h.

Reptiles: 0.01–0.02 mg/kg i.m. q24–48h.

Butorphanol [16]
(Alvegesic, Dolorex, Torbugesic, Torbutrol, Torphasol) POM-V

Formulations:
- Injectable: 10 mg/ml solution.
- Oral: 5 mg, 10 mg tablets.

DOSES

Dogs:
- Analgesia: 0.2–0.5 mg/kg i.v., i.m., s.c.
- Antitussive: 0.05–0.1 mg/kg i.v., i.m., s.c.; 0.5–1 mg/kg p.o q6–12h.

Cats: 0.2–0.5 mg/kg i.v., i.m., s.c.

Small mammals:
- Ferrets: 0.25–0.4 mg/kg s.c. q4–6h.
- Rabbits: 0.1–0.5 mg/kg s.c. q4h.
- Chinchilla: 0.5–2 mg/kg s.c. q4h.
- Guinea pigs: 0.2–2 mg/kg s.c. q4h.
- Gerbils, Hamsters, Rats, Mice: 1–5 mg/kg s.c. q4h.

Birds: 0.3–4 mg/kg i.m., i.v. q6–12h.

Reptiles: 0.5–1 mg/kg i.m.

NOTES

NOTES

Cabergoline [16]

(Galastop) POM-V

Formulations: Oral: 50 µg/ml solution.

DOSES

Dogs:

- 5 µg (micrograms)/kg p.o. q24h for 4–6 days. Control of aggression-related signs may require dosing for 2 weeks.
- To induce abortion: 15 µg/kg p.o. between days 30 and 42.

Cats: To induce abortion: 15 µg (micrograms)/kg p.o. between days 30 and 42.

Rats: 10–50 µg (micrograms)/kg q12–24h.

Birds: 10–50 µg (micrograms)/kg p.o. q24h.

Carbimazole [16]

(Vidalta) POM-V

Formulations: Oral: 10 mg, 15 mg tablets in a sustained release formulation.

DOSES

Dogs, Cats: Starting dose 15 mg/animal p.o. q24h unless total thyroxine concentrations are <100 nmol/l in which case starting dose is 10 mg p.o. q24h. Adjust dose in 5 mg increments but do not break tablets.

NOTES

Cardiopulmonary–cerebral resuscitation (CPCR)[8]

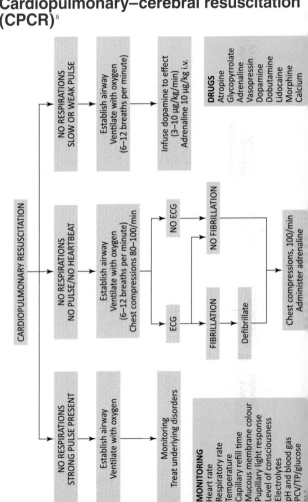

CARDIOPULMONARY RESUSCITATION

NO RESPIRATIONS SLOW OR WEAK PULSE
Establish airway
Ventilate with oxygen (6–12 breaths per minute)
Infuse dopamine to effect (3–10 μg/kg/min)
Adrenaline 10 μg/kg i.v.

NO RESPIRATIONS NO PULSE/NO HEARTBEAT
Establish airway
Ventilate with oxygen (6–12 breaths per minute)
Chest compressions 80–100/min

ECG — FIBRILLATION — Defibrillate
ECG — NO FIBRILLATION
NO ECG — NO FIBRILLATION

Chest compressions, 100/min
Administer adrenaline

NO RESPIRATIONS STRONG PULSE PRESENT
Establish airway
Ventilate with oxygen
Monitoring
Treat underlying disorders

DRUGS
Atropine
Glycopyrrolate
Adrenaline
Vasopressin
Dopamine
Dobutamine
Lidocaine
Morphine
Calcium

MONITORING
Heart rate
Respiratory rate
Temperature
Capillary refill time
Mucous membrane colour
Pupillary light response
Level of consciousness
Electrolytes
pH and blood gas
PCV/TP/glucose

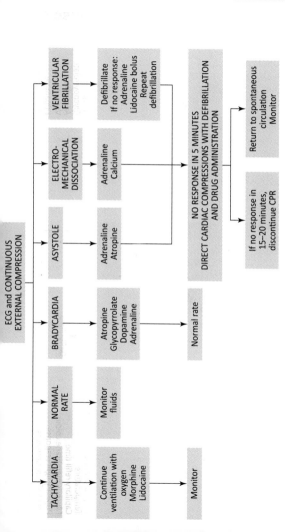

ECG and CONTINUOUS EXTERNAL COMPRESSION

TACHYCARDIA → Continue ventilation with oxygen / Morphine / Lidocaine → Monitor

NORMAL RATE → Monitor fluids

BRADYCARDIA → Atropine / Glycopyrrolate / Dopamine / Adrenaline → Normal rate

ASYSTOLE → Adrenaline / Atropine

ELECTRO-MECHANICAL DISSOCIATION → Adrenaline / Calcium

VENTRICULAR FIBRILLATION → Defibrillate / If no response: Adrenaline / Lidocaine bolus / Repeat defibrillation

NO RESPONSE IN 5 MINUTES
DIRECT CARDIAC COMPRESSIONS WITH DEFIBRILLATION AND DRUG ADMINISTRATION

→ Return to spontaneous circulation / Monitor

→ If no response in 15–20 minutes, discontinue CPR

CPR = cardiopulmonary resuscitation; ECG = electrocardiography; PCV = packed cell volume; TP = total protein.

Carprofen [16]

(Activyl, Bonocarp, Carprieve, Carprodyl, Carprogesic, Dolagis, Norocarp, Norodyl, Rimadyl, Rimifin) POM-V

Formulations:

- Injectable: 50 mg/ml.
- Oral: 20 mg, 50 mg, 100 mg tablets (in plain and palatable formulations).

DOSES

Dogs: 4 mg/kg i.v., s.c. preoperatively or at time of anaesthetic induction; single dose should provide analgesia for up to 24h. Continued analgesia can be provided orally at 4 mg/kg/day, in single or divided dose for up to 5 days after injection. In dogs started on oral medication, subject to clinical response the dose may be reduced to 2 mg/kg/day, single dose, after 7 days.

Carprieve (from datasheet)			
Dose rate	Patient bodyweight (kg)	No. of tablets per dose	
		20 mg	*50 mg*
Dogs			
2 mg/kg once daily	5.0	½	
	10.0	1	
	12.5		½
	15.0	1½	
	20.0	2	
	25.0		1
	37.5		1½
	50.0		2

Cats: 4 mg/kg i.v., s.c., single dose preoperatively or at time of anaesthetic induction.

Small mammals:
- Ferrets: 1 mg/kg p.o.
- Rabbits: 2–4 mg/kg s.c. q24h; 1.5 mg/kg p.o.
- Rodents: 2–5 mg/kg total daily dose i.v., i.m., s.c., p.o., in single or two divided doses.
- Others: 4 mg/kg i.v., i.m., s.c.

Birds: 1–5 mg/kg i.m., s.c., p.o. q12–24h (higher rate appears effective for 24 hours).

Reptiles: 4 mg/kg s.c., i.m., p.o. once, then 2 mg/kg s.c., i.m., p.o. q24h.

Cascade *see* **Prescribing cascade**

NOTES

Cefalexin [16] (Cephalexin)

(Cefaseptin, Cephacare, Ceporex, Rilexine, Therios) POM-V

Formulations:

- Injectable: 180 mg/ml (18%) suspension.
- Oral: 50 mg, 75 mg, 120 mg, 250 mg, 300 mg, 500 mg, 600 mg, 750 mg tablets; granules which, when reconstituted, provide a 100 mg/ml oral syrup.

DOSES

Dogs, Cats: 10–25 mg/kg p.o. q8–12h; i.m, s.c q24h.

Ceporex (from datasheet)				
Dose rate	Patient bodyweight (kg)	No. of tablets per dose, twice daily		
		50 mg tab	*250 mg*	*500 mg*
Dogs				
10–15 mg/kg twice daily for 5 days	≤5	1		
	6–9	2		
	10–25		1	
	26–50		2 or	1
	≥51		3 or	2
Cats				
10–15 mg/kg twice daily for 5 days		1		

Small mammals:

- Ferrets: 15–30 mg/kg p.o. q8–12h.
- Rabbits: 15–20 mg/kg s.c. q12–24h.
- Guinea pigs: 25 mg/kg p.o., i.m q12–24h.
- Others: 15–30 mg/kg i.m. q8–12h.

Birds: 35–100 mg/kg p.o., i.m. q6–8h.

Reptiles: 20–40 mg/kg p.o. q24h at 30°C.

NOTES

Cefovecin [16]

(Convenia) POM-V

Formulations: Injectable: Lyophilized powder which when reconstituted contains 80 mg/ml cefovecin.

DOSES

Dogs, Cats: 8 mg/kg s.c., equivalent to 1 ml/10 kg of reconstituted drug subcutaneously. May be repeated after 14 days up to three times.

Convenia (from datasheet)		
Dose rate	Patient bodyweight (kg)	Volume to be administered (ml)
Dogs and cats		
8 mg/kg (additional doses administered 14 days after first injection)	2.5	0.25
	5	0.5
	10	1.0
	20	2.0
	40	4.0
	60	6.0

Small mammals: Do not use.

Birds: Initial data appear to show it is not practicable (half-life <2h in poultry).

Charcoal [1,16] (Activated charcoal)

(Actidose-Aqua*, Charcodote*, Liqui-Char*) AVM-GSL

Formulations: Oral: 50 g activated charcoal (AC) powder or premixed slurry (200 mg/ml).

- Activated charcoal (AC) should be administered post emesis/ gastric lavage; it acts as an adsorbent for many toxins and further reduces GI absorption.
- Slurries are more effective than tablets or capsules.
- Recommended dose is 1–4 g/kg and may be repeated every 4 to 6 hours for the first 24 to 48 hours or until charcoal is seen in the faeces.
- Repeat dose administration of AC is particularly important when the agent is enterohepatically recirculated, e.g. salicylates, barbiturates, theobromine and methylxanthines.
- AC slows GI transit time, thus co-administration of a cathartic (e.g. sorbitol or magnesium sulphate) can be considered although is not recommended in dehydrated patients or patients where there is a suspicion of ileus.
- AC use may be contraindicated if orally administered treatments or antidotes are to be given.

DOSES

Dogs, Cats: 0.5–4 g/kg as a slurry in water by stomach tube; usually followed by a saline cathartic 20–30 min later.

Small mammals: 0.5–5 g/kg p.o. (anecdotal).

NOTES

Chinchilla biological data[14]

Lifespan (years)	Average 8–10 (maximum 18)
Adult bodyweight (g)	Males: 450–600 Females: 550–800 (females are usually larger than males)
Dentition	2 [I 1/1, C0/0, P1/1, M3/3]
Body temperature (°C)	37–38
Heart rate (beats/min)	200–350
Respiratory rate (breaths/min)	40–80
Tidal volume (ml/kg)	Not found in the literature
Food consumption	21 g/day (adult); eat with forefeet
Water consumption	45–70 ml/day, depending on moisture content of food
Sexual maturity (months)	6–8
Oestrous cycle	40 days; seasonally polyoestrous (November to May)
Duration of oestrus	3–5 days
Gestation length (days)	111
Parturition	Early morning; does not usually nest
Post-partum oestrus	Yes
Litter size	1–6 (average 2)
Birth weight (g)	30–50; precocial; fully furred; active
Eyes open (days)	Open at birth
Eat solid food (days)	May begin day after birth to nibble solid foods

Chlorphenamine [16] (Chlorpheniramine)
(Piriton*) POM, GSL

Formulations:

- Injectable: 10 mg/ml solution.
- Oral: 4 mg tablet, 0.4 mg/ml syrup.

DOSES

Dogs: 4–8 mg/dog p.o. q8h; 2.5–10 mg/dog i.m. or slow i.v.

Cats: 2–4 mg/cat p.o. q8–12h; 2–5 mg/cat i.m. or slow i.v.

Small mammals:

- Ferrets: 1–2 mg/kg p.o. q8–12h.
- Rabbits: 0.2–0.4 mg/kg p.o. q12h.
- Rodents: 0.6 mg/kg p.o. q24h.

NOTES

Clindamycin [16]

(Antirobe, Clindacin, Clindacyl) POM-V

Formulations: Oral: 25 mg, 75 mg, 150 mg, 300 mg capsules.

DOSES

Dogs: 5.5 mg/kg p.o. q12h or 11 mg/kg q24h; in severe infection can increase to 11 mg/kg q12h.

- Toxoplasmosis: 25 mg/kg p.o. daily in divided doses.

Cats: 5.5 mg/kg p.o. q12h or 11mg/kg q24h.

- Toxoplasmosis: 25 mg/kg p.o. daily in divided doses.

Antirobe, Clindacin, Clindacyl (from datasheet)					
Dose rate	Patient bodyweight (kg)	No. of tablets required			
		25 mg	*75 mg*	*150 mg*	*300 mg*
Dogs and cats					
5.5 mg/kg q12h	4.5	1, twice daily			
	13.5		1, twice daily		
	27			1, twice daily	
11 mg/kg q24h	4.5	2, once daily			
	13.5			1, once daily	
	27				1, once daily
11 mg/kg q12h	4.5	2, twice daily			
	13.5			1, twice daily	
	27				1, twice daily

➡

Small mammals:
- Ferrets: 5.5–11 mg/kg p.o. q12h (toxoplasmosis: 12.5–25 mg/kg p.o. q12h).
- Rabbits, Rodents: *Do not use*.

Birds: 25 mg/kg p.o. q8h or 50 mg/kg p.o. q12h or 100 mg/kg p.o. q24h.

Reptiles: 2.5–5 mg/kg p.o. q24h.

Clotting factor tests[8]

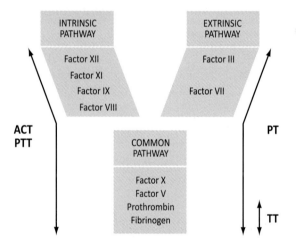

Factors evaluated with the screening coagulation tests.

ACT = activated clotting time; PTT = partial thromboplastin time; PT = prothrombin time; TT = thrombin time.

NOTES

Collapse – emergency evaluation[8]

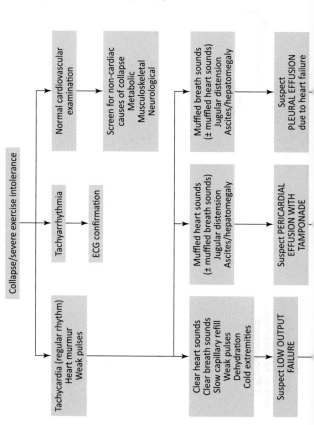

Collapse/severe exercise intolerance

Tachycardia (regular rhythm) / Heart murmur / Weak pulses

- Clear heart sounds, Clear breath sounds, Slow capillary refill, Weak pulses, Dehydration, Cold extremities → Suspect LOW OUTPUT FAILURE

- Muffled heart sounds (± muffled breath sounds), Jugular distension, Ascites/hepatomegaly → Suspect PERICARDIAL EFFUSION WITH TAMPONADE

Tachyarrhythmia → ECG confirmation

Normal cardiovascular examination → Screen for non-cardiac causes of collapse: Metabolic, Musculoskeletal, Neurological

- Muffled breath sounds (± muffled heart sounds), Jugular distension, Ascites/hepatomegaly → Suspect PLEURAL EFFUSION due to heart failure

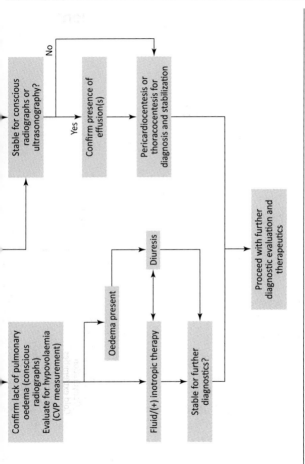

CVP = central venous pressure; ECG = electrocardiography.

NOTES

CPCR *see* Cardiopulmonary–cerebral resuscitation

Cranial draw test[3]

Indications/Use

- To diagnose partial or complete rupture of the cranial cruciate ligament (CCL)
- Note: this test does *not* identify isolated rupture of the caudomedial band of the CCL
- Often used in association with the tibial compression test

Contraindications

Periarticular fibrosis and meniscal injury, with the caudal horn of the medial meniscus wedged between the femoral condyle and tibial plateau, may prevent cranial draw in a CCL-deficient stifle

Patient preparation and positioning

- Can be performed in the conscious animal. However, if the patient is tense (due to pain or temperament) or if the CCL is only partially torn, sedation or general anaesthesia may be required.
- A conscious patient may be restrained in a standing position on three legs, with the affected limb held off the ground.
- Sedated or anaesthetized patients may be positioned in lateral recumbency, with the affected limb uppermost.

Technique

1. Grasp the distal femur in one hand, placing the thumb over the lateral fabella and the index finger on the patella.
2. Use the other hand to grasp the proximal tibia, placing the thumb over the head of the fabella and the index finger on the tibial crest.
3. Apply a cranial force to the tibia while the stifle joint is held in full extension, and then while the joint is held in 30–60 degrees of flexion.

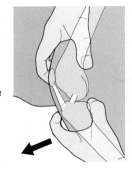

Results

- Complete rupture of the CCL is associated with cranial displacement of the tibia relative to the femur, in both *extension and flexion*.
- Isolated rupture of the *craniomedial* band of the CCL is associated with cranial displacement of the tibia relative to the femur, in *flexion* only.
- A short cranial draw motion, with a sharp end point, may be detected in young animals and is normal.

See also Tibial compression test

Cranial nerve numbering[11]

CN I	Olfactory nerve		CN VII	Facial nerve
CN II	Optic nerve		CN VIII	Vestibulocochlear nerve
CN III	Oculomotor nerve		CN IX	Glossopharyngeal nerve
CN IV	Trochlear nerve		CN X	Vagus nerve
CN V	Trigeminal nerve		CN XI	Accessory nerve
CN VI	Abducent nerve		CN XII	Hypoglossal nerve

Cranial nerve tests [11]

Cranial nerve test	Afferent cranial nerve	Intermediate brain region	Efferent cranial nerve	Principal effect noted
Palpebral reflex	CN V – Trigeminal (ophthalmic or maxillary)	Brainstem	CN VII – Facial	Blink elicited by touching of the medial or lateral canthus of the eye
Corneal sensation	CN V – Trigeminal (ophthalmic)	Brainstem	CN VII – Facial CN VI – Abducent	Blink and globe retraction elicited by touching the cornea
Vestibulo-ocular reflex	CN VIII – Vestibulocochlear	Brainstem	CN III – Oculomotor CN IV – Trochlear CN VI – Abducent	Nystagmus induced by moving the head
Menace response	CN II – Optic	Forebrain Cerebellum Brainstem	CN VII – Facial	Blink elicited by a menacing gesture
Response to stimulation of nasal mucosa	CN V – Trigeminal (ophthalmic)	Forebrain Brainstem	None	Withdrawal of the head elicited by touching the nasal mucosa
Pupillary light reflex	CN II – Optic	Brainstem	CN III – Oculomotor	Pupillary constriction elicited by shining a light in the eye
Gag reflex	CN IX – Glossopharyngeal CN X – Vagus	Brainstem	CN IX – Glossopharyngeal CN X – Vagus	Contraction of the pharynx elicited by its palpation

NOTES

NOTES

NOTES

NOTES

Degu biological data [14]

Lifespan (years)	7–10
Adult bodyweight (g)	176–315
Dentition	2 [I 1/1, C0/0, P1/1, M3/3]
Body temperature (°C)	36.8–37.6
Heart rate (beats/min)	Not published
Respiratory rate (breaths/min)	Not published
Tidal volume (ml/kg)	Not found in the literature
Food consumption	10.2–15.1 g/day (non-breeding adult)
Water consumption	10.3–40.4 ml/day, depending on moisture content of food
Sexual maturity (months)	6 (range: 45 days to 20 months)
Oestrous cycle	No regular oestrous cycle; presence of male may be needed to induce ovulation; breed all year in captivity
Duration of oestrus	Receptive for several hours; multiple copulations
Gestation length (days)	90–93
Parturition	Early morning; does not usually nest
Post-partum oestrus	No
Litter size	5–6 (1–10 per litter possible)
Birth weight (g)	14.1–14.6 g; precocial; fully furred; active
Eyes open (days)	Open at birth
Eat solid food (days)	May begin day after birth to nibble solid foods

Delmadinone[16]

(Tardak) POM-V

Formulations: Injectable: 10 mg/ml suspension.

DOSES

Dogs: 1.5–2 mg/kg (dogs <10 kg); 1–1.5 mg/kg (10–20 kg); 1 mg/kg (>20 kg) i.m., s.c. repeated after 8 days if no response. Animals that respond to treatment may need further treatment after 3–4 weeks.

Cats: 1.5 mg/kg repeated after 8 days if no response. Animals that respond to treatment may need further treatment after 3–4 weeks.

Birds: 1 mg/kg i.m. once.

Dexamethasone[16]

(Aurizon, Dexadreson, Dexafort, Rapidexon, Voren, Maxidex*, Maxitrol*) POM-V

Formulations:
- Ophthalmic: 0.1% solution (Maxidex, Maxitrol). Maxitrol also contains polymyxin B and neomycin.
- Injectable: 2 mg/ml solution; 1 mg/ml, 3 mg/ml suspensions; 2.5 mg/ml suspension with 7.5 mg/ml prednisolone.
- Oral: 0.5 mg tablet.
- (1 mg of dexamethasone is equivalent to 1.1 mg of dexamethasone acetate, 1.3 mg of dexamethasone isonicotinate or dexamethasone sodium phosphate, or 1.4 mg of dexamethasone trioxa-undecanoate.)

DOSES

Dogs:
- Ophthalmic: Apply small amount of ointment to affected eye(s) q6–24h or 1 drop of solution in affected eye(s) q6–12h.
- Cerebral oedema: 2–3 mg/kg i.v., then 1 mg/kg s.c. q6–8h, taper off.
- Inflammation: 0.01–0.16 mg/kg i.m., s.c., p.o. q24h for 3–5 days maximum.
- Prevention and treatment of anaphylaxis: 0.5 mg/kg i.v. once.

- Immunosuppression: 0.3–0.64 mg/kg i.m., s.c., p.o. q24h for up to 5 days.
- Assessment of adrenal function: low dose dexamethasone suppression test (0.015 mg/kg i.v.).

Cats:

- Ophthalmic, Cerebral oedema, Inflammation, Anaphylaxis, Immunosuppression: doses as for dogs.
- Assessment of adrenal function: dexamethasone suppression test (0.15 mg/kg i.v.). *NB: note difference to dogs.*

Small mammals:

- Ferrets: 0.5–2.0 mg/kg s.c., i.m., i.v. q24h.
- Rabbits: 0.2–0.6 mg/kg s.c., i.m., i.v. q24h.
- Others: anti-inflammatory: 0.05–0.2 mg/kg i.m., s.c. q12–24h tapering dose over 3–14 days.

Birds: 2–6 mg/kg i.v., i.m. q12–24h.

Reptiles: Inflammatory, non-infectious respiratory disease: 2–4 mg/kg i.m., i.v. q24h for 3 days.

Dexmedetomidine [16]

(Dexdomitor) POM-V

Formulations: Injectable: 0.5 mg/ml solution.

DOSES

Dogs, Cats: Premedication: 3–5 µg (micrograms)/kg i.v., i.m, s.c. in combination with an opioid (use lower end of dose range i.v.).

See also **Premedication protocols – drug combinations used in dogs and cats *and* Sedation combinations**

NOTES

Diazepam [16]

(Diazemuls*, Diazepam*, Diazepam Rectubes*, Valium*) POM

Formulations:

- Injectable: 5 mg/ml emulsion (Diazemuls), 5 mg/ml diazepam in propylene glycol.
- Oral: 2 mg, 5 mg, 10 mg tablets; 2 mg/5 ml solution.
- Rectal: 2 mg/ml (1.25, 2.5 ml tubes); 10 mg suppositories.

DOSES

Dogs:

- Anxiolytic: 0.5–2.0 mg/kg p.o as required.
- Skeletal muscle relaxation: 2–10 mg/dog p.o. q8h.
- Emergency management of seizures, including status epilepticus: bolus dose of 0.5–1 mg/kg i.v. or intrarectally (if venous access is not available). Time to onset of clinical effect is 2–3 min for i.v. use; therefore repeat every 10 min if no clinical effect, up to three times. Additional doses may be administered if appropriate supportive care facilities are available (for support of respiration). Constant rate i.v. infusion for control of status epilepticus or cluster seizures: initial rate 1 mg/kg/h, may be titrated upwards to effect.

Cats:

- Anxiolytic: 0.2–0.4 mg/kg p.o. q8h.
- Appetite stimulant: 0.5–1.0 mg/kg i.v. once.
- Behavioural modification of urine spraying and muscle relaxation: 1.25–5 mg/cat p.o. q8h. The dose should be gradually increased to achieve the desired effect without concurrent sedation.
- Emergency management of seizures including status epilepticus: bolus dose of 0.5–1 mg/kg i.v. or intrarectally if venous access is not available. Time to onset of clinical effect is 2–3 min for i.v. use, therefore repeat every 10 min if there is no clinical effect, up to maximum of three times. Constant rate i.v. infusion for the control of status epilepticus or cluster seizures: initial rate of 0.5 mg/kg/h. *Care should be taken in cats to avoid overdosing: if cats demonstrate excessive sedation then diazepam should be discontinued.*

Small mammals:

- Ferrets: seizures: 2–5 mg/kg i.m. once.
- Rabbits: epileptic seizures: 1 mg/kg i.v. once.
- Guinea pigs: 0.5–5.0 mg/kg i.m. once.
- Chinchillas, Hamsters, Gerbils, Rats, Mice: 2.5–5 mg/kg i.m., i.p. once.

Birds:

- Epileptic seizures: 0.1–1 mg/kg i.v., i.m. once.
- Appetite stimulant in raptors: 0.2 mg/kg p.o. q24h.

Reptiles: Epileptic seizures: 2.5 mg/kg i.m., i.v. once.

Diltiazem [16]

(Hypercard, Dilcardia SR*) POM-V, POM

Formulations: Oral: 10 mg (Hypercard), 60 mg (generic) tablets. Long-acting preparations authorized for humans, such as Dilcardia SR (60 mg, 90 mg, 120 mg capsules), are available but their pharmacokinetics have been little studied in animals to date.

DOSES

Long-acting preparations have been used at a dose of 10 mg/kg p.o. q24h but there is little experience with such formulations in animals.

Dogs: 0.05–0.25 mg/kg i.v. over 1–2 minutes, 0.5–2.0 mg/kg p.o. q8h. Lower doses are preferred in the presence of heart failure.

Cats: 0.05–0.25 mg/kg i.v. over 1–2 minutes, 0.5–2.5 mg/kg p.o. q8h, or one 10 mg tablet for cats of 3–6.25 kg p.o. q8h.

Small mammals: Ferrets: 1.5–7.5 mg/kg p.o. q12h.

Doxapram [16]

(Dopram-V) POM-VPS, POM-V

Formulations:

- Injectable: 20 mg/ml solution.
- Oral: 20 mg/ml drops.

Dogs, Cats: 5–10 mg/kg i.v., repeat according to need.
- Neonates: 1–2 drops under the tongue (oral solution) or 0.1 ml i.v. into the umbilical vein; this should be used once only.

Small mammals:
- Ferrets, Rabbits, Chinchillas, Hamsters, Gerbils, Rats, Mice: 5–10 mg/kg i.v., i.m., i.p., sublingual once
- Guinea pigs: 2–5 mg/kg i.v., s.c., i.p. once.

Birds: 5–20 mg/kg i.m., i.v., intratracheal, intraosseous once.

Reptiles: 4–12 mg/kg i.m., i.v., p.o. once.

Doxycycline [16]
(Doxyseptin 300, Ornicure, Pulmodox, Ronaxan, Vibramycin*, Vibravenos*) POM-V

Formulations:
- Oral: 20 mg, 100 mg tablets (Ronaxan); 300 mg tablets (Doxyseptin); 260 mg/sachet powder (Ornicure).
- Injectable: 20 mg/ml long-acting injection (Vibravenos; import on a Special Treatment Certificate).

Dogs, Cats: 10 mg/kg p.o. q24h with food.
- Feline chlamydophilosis: 5 mg/kg p.o. q12h for 3 weeks.

Small mammals:
- Rabbits: 2.5–4 mg/kg p.o. q24h.
- Rats, Mice: 5 mg/kg p.o. q12h.
- Other rodents: 2.5 mg/kg p.o. q12h.

Birds:
- Parrots: 15–50 mg/kg p.o. q24h, 1000 mg/kg in soft food/dehulled seed, 75–100 mg/kg i.m. q7d (Vibravenos; lowest dose rate for macaws); course of treatment with doxycycline for chlamydophilosis = 45 days.
- Raptors: 50 mg/kg p.o. q12h, 100 mg/kg i.m. q7d (Vibravenos).
- Passerines/Pigeons: 40 mg/kg p.o. 12–24h, 200–500 mg/l in water (soft or deionized water only).

Reptiles: 50 mg/kg i.m. once, then 25 mg/kg i.m. q72h.

Drug distribution categories [16]

AVM-GSL: Authorized veterinary medicine – general sales list (formerly GSL). This may be sold by anyone.

NFA-VPS: Non-food animal medicine – veterinarian, pharmacist, Suitably Qualified Person (SQP) (formerly PML companion animal products and a few P products). These medicines for companion animals must be supplied by a veterinary surgeon, pharmacist or SQP. An SQP has to be registered with the Animal Medicines Training Regulatory Authority (AMTRA). Veterinary nurses can become SQPs but it is not automatic.

POM-VPS: Prescription-only medicine – veterinarian, pharmacist, SQP (formerly PML livestock products, MFSX products and a few P products). These medicines for food-producing animals (including horses) can only be supplied on an oral or written veterinary prescription from a veterinary surgeon, pharmacist or SQP and can only be supplied by one of those groups of people in accordance with the prescription.

POM-V: Prescription-only medicine – veterinarian (formerly POM products and a few P products). These medicines can only be supplied against a veterinary prescription that has been prepared (either orally or in writing) by a veterinary surgeon to animals under their care following a clinical assessment, and can only be supplied by a veterinary surgeon or pharmacist in accordance with the prescription.

ZFA: This non-official term is used to indicate a zootechnical feed additive.

SAES: This non-official term is used to indicate medicines marketed in accordance with the Small Animal Exemption Scheme.

CD: Controlled Drug. A substance controlled by the Misuse of Drugs Act 1971 and Regulations. The CD is followed by (Schedule 1), (Schedule 2), (Schedule 3), (Schedule 4) or (Schedule 5).

NOTES

NOTES

NOTES

NOTES

ECG standard leads, lead II diagram and reference ranges [15]

The animal should be placed in right lateral recumbency.

Standard leads for electrocardiography

Lead	Attachment site	Colour
RA (right 'arm')	Right elbow	Red
LA (left 'arm')	Left elbow	Yellow
F or LL (left leg)	Left stifle	Green
N or RL (right leg, earth lead)	Right stifle	Black

Lead II at 1 cm/mV and 50 mm/s

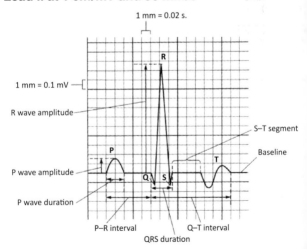

Reference ranges

Parameter	Unit	Dogs	Cats
Heart rate	beats per minute	70–160 for adult dogs 60–140 for giant breeds up to 180 for toy breeds up to 220 for puppies	120–240
P wave duration	seconds	<0.04 (<0.05 in giant breeds)	<0.04
P wave amplitude	mV	<0.4	<0.2
P–R interval	seconds	0.06–0.13	0.05–0.09
QRS duration	seconds	<0.06	<0.04
R wave amplitude	mV	<2.5–3.0	<0.9
Q–T interval	seconds	0.15–0.25	0.12–0.18
Mean electrical axis (MEA)	degrees	+40 to +100	0 to +160

Data from Tilley LP (1992) *Essentials of Canine and Feline Electrocardiography: Interpretation and Management, 3rd edition*. Philadelphia, Lea & Febiger

NOTES

Ectoparasite treatments [2]

Host species	Minimum age for first use	Spectrum of activity			
		Fleas	Biting lice	Flies	Ticks
Trade name: ADVANTAGE **Active ingredient:** Imidacloprid **Presentation:** Spot-on					
C,D,R	8 weeks: C,D *** 10 weeks: R	✓ A,L	✓ D only		
Trade name: ADVANTIX **Active ingredients:** Imidacloprid, Permethrin **Presentation:** Spot-on					
D	7 weeks **	✓ A		Mosquito Sandfly Stablefly	✓
Trade name: ADVOCATE **Active ingredients:** Imidacloprid, Moxidectin **Presentation:** Spot-on					
C,D,F	9 weeks: C 7 weeks: D	✓ A	✓ D only		
Trade name: ALUDEX **Active ingredient:** Amitraz **Presentation:** Emulsion for external use only					
D	12 weeks				
Trade name: CAPSTAR **Active ingredient:** Nitenpyram **Presentation:** Tablet					
C,D	4 weeks **	✓ A			
Trade name: CERTIFECT **Active ingredients:** Fipronil, Amitraz, S-Methoprene **Presentation:** Spot-on					
D	8 weeks **	✓ A,L,O	✓		✓

Host species: C = cat, D = dog, F = ferret, R = rabbit.
Action: A = Adulticidal, L = larvicidal, O = ovaricidal.

* Can be used in pregnant bitches/queens.
** Can be used during pregnancy and lactation.
*** Can be used in nursing bitches/queens.

Demodex	Sarcoptes	Ear mites	Endopara-sites	Affected by weekly bath/swim	Frequency of use
				✓	4 weeks
				✓	4 weeks
✓ D only	✓ D only	✓ C,D	Di: C,D,F Av & Cv: D Tc, At: C,D Tv, Tl, Us: D	✓	4 weeks
✓	✓			✓	Weekly
				✗	Use with other
				✓	Every 2 weeks max.

Endoparasites: *At* = *Ancylostoma tubaeforme*, *Av* = *Angiostrongylus vasorum*, *Cv* = *Crenosoma vulpis*, *Di* = *Dirofilaria immitis*, *Tc* = *Toxocara cati/canis*, *Tl* = *Toxascaris leonina*, *Tv* = *Trichuris vulpis*, *Us* = *Uncinaria stenocephala*.

Host species	Minimum age for first use	Spectrum of activity			
		Fleas	Biting lice	Flies	Ticks
Trade name: COMFORTIS **Active ingredient:** Spinosad **Presentation:** Tablet					
D	14 weeks	✓ A,O			
Trade name: EFFIPRO **Active ingredient:** Fipronil **Presentation:** Spot-on, Spray					
C,D	8 weeks 2 days	✓ A ✓ A	✗ ✓		✓ ✓
Trade name: FRONTLINE COMBO **Active ingredients:** Fipronil, S-methoprene **Presentation:** Spot-on					
C,D	8 weeks **	✓ A,L,O	✓		✓
Trade name: FRONTLINE 4FLEAS FIPRONIL **Active ingredient:** Fipronil **Presentation:** Spot-on, Spray					
C,D C,D	8 weeks ** 2 days	✓ A ✓ A	✓ ✓		✓ ✓
Trade name: FIPROCAT FIPROLINE FOR CATS **Active ingredient:** Fipronil **Presentation:** Spot-on					
C	8 weeks	✓ A			
Trade name: FIPRODOG FIPROLINE FOR DOGS **Active ingredient:** Fipronil **Presentation:** Spot-on					
D	8 weeks	✓ A			(✓)
Trade name: FIPROSPOT **Active ingredient:** Fipronil **Presentation:** Spot-on					
C,D	8 weeks	✓ A			(✓) D
Trade name: PRAC-TIC **Active ingredient:** Pyriprole **Presentation:** Spot-on					
D	8 weeks	✓ A,O			✓

Host species: C = cat, D = dog, F = ferret, R = rabbit.
Action: A = Adulticidal, L = larvicidal, O = ovaricidal.

* Can be used in pregnant bitches/queens.
** Can be used during pregnancy and lactation.
*** Can be used in nursing bitches/queens.

Demodex	Sarcoptes	Ear mites	Endopara-sites	Affected by weekly bath/swim	Frequency of use
				X	4 weeks
				X	4 weeks
				X	4 weeks
				X	4 weeks
				X	4 weeks
				X	4 weeks
				X	4 weeks
				X	4 weeks
				X	4 weeks

Endoparasites: At = Ancylostoma tubaeforme, Av = Angiostrongylus vasorum, Cv = Crenosoma vulpis, Di = Dirofilaria immitis, Tc = Toxocara cati/canis, Tl = Toxascaris leonina, Tv = Trichuris vulpis, Us = Uncinaria stenocephala.

Host species	Minimum age for first use	Spectrum of activity			
		Fleas	Biting lice	Flies	Ticks
Trade name: PROGRAM **Active ingredient:** Lufenuron **Presentation:** Tablet, Suspension, Injectable					
D C	Puppies/ kittens taking solid food *	✓ L,O			
Trade name: PROGRAM PLUS **Active ingredients:** Lufenuron, Milbemycin oxime **Presentation:** Tablet					
D		✓ L,O			
Trade name: PROMERIS **Active ingredient:** Metaflumizone **Presentation:** Spot-on					
C	8 weeks**	✓ A			
Trade name: PROMERIS DUO **Active ingredients:** Metaflumizone, Amitraz **Presentation:** Spot-on					
D	8 weeks**	✓ A	✓	✓	✓
Trade name: SCALIBOR **Active ingredient:** Deltamethrin **Presentation:** Collar					
D	7 weeks**			Mosquito Sandflies	✓
Trade name: STRONGHOLD **Active ingredient:** Selamectin **Presentation:** Spot-on					
C,D	6 weeks**	✓ A,L,O	✓		

Host species: C = cat, D = dog, F = ferret, R = rabbit.
Action: A = Adulticidal, L = larvicidal, O = ovaricidal.

* Can be used in pregnant bitches/queens.
** Can be used during pregnancy and lactation.
*** Can be used in nursing bitches/queens.

Demodex	Sarcoptes	Ear mites	Endoparasites	Affected by weekly bath/swim	Frequency of use
				✗	4 weeks
			Di, Ac, Tc, Tv	✗	4 weeks
				✓	4 weeks
✓				✓	4 weeks
				✓	5–6 months
	✓ D only	✓	Di, Tc At: C only	✗	4 weeks

Endoparasites: At = Ancylostoma tubaeforme, Av = Angiostrongylus vasorum, Cv = Crenosoma vulpis, Di = Dirofilaria immitis, Tc = Toxocara cati/canis, Tl = Toxascaris leonina, Tv = Trichuris vulpis, Us = Uncinaria stenocephala.

See also Fipronil, Imidacloprid, Lufenuron, Methoprene, Moxidectin *and* Selamectin

Emergency drug doses *see page 214*

Emesis induction[1]

Contraindications to the induction of emesis include:

- The ingested substance is caustic, acidic, volatile, petroleum- or detergent-based
- The patient has severe CNS depression
- The patient has respiratory distress
- The poison ingested is known to cause seizures.

Remember that some emetics have a short delay before action.

Emetics cannot be used in horses, rodents, rabbits or ruminants.

There are several options for the induction of emesis:

- Apomorphine – may be given by the intravenous, intramuscular, subcutaneous or conjunctival route. The dose is 0.02–0.04 mg/kg and the route chosen will depend on the preparation available. It is a centrally acting emetic that is extremely effective in dogs but is not recommended in cats as it is variably effective
- Alpha-2 agonists (e.g. xylazine, medetomidine) – effective emetics in cats but not useful in dogs. The sedative effects may be unwelcome. They are more effective if the cat's stomach is full
- Sodium carbonate (washing soda) crystals – an effective emetic in dogs and cats. The dose is empirical but usually a large crystal in a medium- to large-breed dog and a small crystal in a small dog or cat is sufficient. Although it may be administered by the owner, caution is recommended as it is mildly caustic. It is also vital that it is not confused with caustic soda (sodium hydroxide)!
- Other options such as Syrup of Ipecac, household remedies (table salt, mustard) and hydrogen peroxide are *not recommended* and can be dangerous.

Enrofloxacin [16]

(Baytril, Enrocare, Enrotab, Enrox, Enroxil, Floxabactin, Floxibac, Powerflox, Xeden) POM-V

Formulations:

- Injectable: 25 mg/ml, 50 mg/ml, 100 mg/ml solutions.
- Oral: 15 mg, 50 mg, 150 mg tablets; 25 mg/ml solution.

DOSES

Dogs, Cats: 5 mg/kg s.c., i.v. q24h; 2.5 mg/kg p.o. q12h or 5 mg/kg p.o. q24h. Some isolates of *Pseudomonas aeruginosa* may require higher doses, contact the manufacturer to discuss individual cases.

Baytril Flavour Tablets (from datasheet)				
Dose rate	No. of tablets per total daily dose			
	15 mg	*50 mg*	*150 mg*	*250 mg*
Cats and small dogs				
5 mg/kg once daily or as a divided dose twice daily for 3 to 10 days	1 per 3 kg bodyweight			
Medium dogs				
5 mg/kg once daily or as a divided dose twice daily for 3 to 10 days		1 per 10 kg bodyweight		
Large dogs				
5 mg/kg once daily or as a divided dose twice daily for 3 to 10 days			1 per 30 kg bodyweight	1 per 50 kg bodyweight

Small mammals:
- Ferrets: 5–10 mg/kg p.o., s.c., i.m. q12h or 10–20 mg/kg p.o., s.c., i.m. q24h.
- Rabbits: 10–30 mg/kg p.o., s.c., i.v. q24h.
- Rodents: 5–10 mg/kg s.c., p.o. q12–24h.
- Others: 5–10 mg/kg s.c., p.o. q12h or 20 mg/kg s.c., p.o. q24h.

Birds: 10–15 mg/kg i.m., p.o. q12h (sensitive infections can be treated q24h) or 100–200 mg/l drinking water.

Reptiles: 5–10 mg/kg i.m., p.o. q24–48h.

NOTES

NOTES

NOTES

Fenbendazole [16]

(Bob Martin Easy to Use Wormer, Granofen, Lapizole, Panacur, Zerofen) NFA-VPS

Formulations: Oral: 222 mg/g granules (22%); 20 mg/ml (2%), 25 mg/ml (2.5%), 100 mg/ml (10%) suspensions; 0.187 g/g paste in a syringe; 500 mg, 1000 mg chewable tablets; 8 mg capsule (for pigeons).

DOSES

Dogs:

- Roundworms, tapeworms: dogs <6 months old: 50 mg/kg p.o. q24h for 3 consecutive days; >6 months old, 100 mg/kg as a single dose p.o. Treatment of *Capillaria* may need to be extended to 10 days. Repeat q3months. For pregnant bitches 25 mg/kg p.o. q24h from day 40 until 2 days post-whelping (approximately 25 days).
- *Angiostrongylus vasorum*, *Oslerus osleri*: 50 mg/kg p.o. q24h for 7 days.
- Giardiasis: 50 mg/kg p.o. q24h for 3 days.

Cats:

- Roundworms, tapeworms: cats <6 months old: 20 mg/kg p.o. q24h for 5 days; >6 months old, 100 mg/kg as a single dose p.o.
- *Aelurostrongylus abstrusus*: 20 mg/kg p.o. q24h for 5 days.
- Giardiasis: 20 mg/kg p.o. for 5 days.

Panacur (from datasheet)		
Dose rate	**Patient bodyweight**	**Volume required**
2.5% ORAL SUSPENSION		
Adult dogs and cats		
100 mg/kg or 4 ml/kg	250 g	1 ml
	500 g	2 ml
	750 g	3 ml
	1 kg	4 ml
	1.5 kg	6 ml
	2 kg	8 ml
	2.5 kg	10 ml

Panacur (from datasheet)

Dose rate	Patient bodyweight	Volume required
Puppies and kittens under 6 months of age		
50 mg/kg or 2 ml/kg daily for 3 consecutive days	250 g	0.5 ml daily for 3 days
	500 g	1 ml daily for 3 days
	1 kg	2 ml daily for 3 days
	1.5 kg	3 ml daily for 3 days
	2 kg	4 ml daily for 3 days
Pregnant dogs		
25 mg/kg or 1 ml/kg (from day 40 of pregnancy continuously to 2 days post-whelping)	2–4 kg	4 ml daily for approx. 25 days
	4–8 kg	8 ml daily for approx. 25 days
	8–16 kg	16 ml daily for approx. 25 days
10% ORAL SUSPENSION		
Adult dogs and cats		
100 mg/kg or 1 ml/kg	2–4 kg	4 ml
	4–8 kg	8 ml
	8–16 kg	16 ml
	16–24 kg	24 ml
	24–32 kg	32 ml
	32–64 kg	64 ml
Puppies and kittens under 6 months of age		
50 mg/kg or 0.5 ml/kg daily for 3 consecutive days	<1 kg	0.5 ml daily for 3 days
	1–2 kg	1 ml daily for 3 days
	2–4 kg	2 ml daily for 3 days
	4–6 kg	3 ml daily for 3 days
	6–8 kg	4 ml daily for 3 days
	8–10 kg	5 ml daily for 3 days
Pregnant dogs		
25 mg/kg or 1 ml/4 kg (from day 40 of pregnancy continuously to 2 days post-whelping)	4 kg	1 ml daily for approx 25 days
	8 kg	2 ml daily for approx 25 days
	12 kg	3 ml daily for approx 25 days
	20 kg	5 ml daily for approx 25 days
	40 kg	10 ml daily for approx 25 days

Small mammals:

- Rabbits: *Encephalitozoon cuniculi*: 20 mg/kg p.o. q24h for 28 days.
- Other small mammals: 20–50 mg/kg p.o. q24h for 5 consecutive days; the higher end of the range is suggested for giardiasis only.

Birds:

- Nematodes: 20–100 mg/kg p.o., administer 2 doses separated by 10 days; capillariasis: 25 mg/kg p.o. q24h for 5 consecutive days. Pigeons: 16 mg/kg p.o. once, repeat after 10 days if necessary or 10–20 mg/kg p.o. q24h for 3 days, repeat after 2 weeks. Passerines: 20 mg/kg p.o. q24h for 3 doses. Not advisable to give more than 50 mg/kg in unfamiliar species.
- Giardiasis: 50 mg/kg p.o. q24h for 3 doses.

Reptiles:

- Nematodes: 50–100 mg/kg once p.o., per cloaca; repeat after 2 and 4 weeks.
- Giardiasis and flagellates: 50 mg/kg p.o. q24h for 3–5 days. In species with potential toxicity, e.g. ball pythons (*Python regius*): 25 mg/kg p.o.

NOTES

Ferret biological data[14]

Lifespan (years)	8–10 (max. 15); 5–7 in the USA
Average bodyweight (g)	Males: 1200 Females: 600
Rectal temperature (°C)	38.8 (37.8–40)
Heart rate (beats/min)	200–250
Respiration rate (breaths/min)	33–36
Sexual maturity	First Spring after birth
Breeding season	Northern hemisphere: March–September Southern hemisphere: August–January
Gestation period	41–42 days
Average litter size	8
Weight at birth	8–10 g
Eyes open at	4–5 weeks
Eruption of deciduous teeth	3–4 weeks
Eruption of permanent teeth	7–10 weeks
Weaning age	6–8 weeks (preferably 8)

Fipronil[16]
(4 Fleas, Effipro, Fiproline, Frontline, Frontline Combo, Vexitor)
NFA-VPS

Formulations: Topical: 10% w/v fipronil spot-on pipettes in a wide range of sizes (4Fleas, Effipro, Fiproline, Frontline, Vexitor); with *S*-methoprene (Frontline Combo). Also 0.25% w/v fipronil spray in alcohol base (Effipro, Fiproline and Frontline sprays) in a range of sizes.

DOSES

Dogs:
- Flea infestations: spray 3–6 ml/kg (6–12 pumps/kg 100 ml application, 2–4 pumps/kg 250 ml or 500 ml application) or apply 1 pipette per dog according to body weight. Treatment should be repeated not more frequently than every 4 weeks.

■ Cheyletiellosis, Otocariosis (*Otodectes cynotis*): same dose but for two applications.

Cats: Spray 3–6 ml/kg (6–12 pumps/kg 100 ml application) or apply 1 pipette per cat. Treatment should be repeated not more frequently than every 4 weeks.

Small mammals:
■ Ferrets: spray 3–6 ml/kg q30–60d.
■ Rodents: 7.5 mg/kg topically q30–60d.

Birds: Use spray form q30–60d. Apply to cotton wool and dab behind head, under wings and at base of tail (raptors/parrots) or lightly under each wing (pigeon/passerine).

Reptiles: Spray on to cloth first then wipe over surface of reptile q7–14d until negative for ectoparasites.

Firocoxib [16]
(Previcox) POM-V

Formulations: Oral: 57 mg, 227 mg tablets.

DOSES

Dogs: 5 mg/kg p.o. q24h, with or without food.

Previcox (from datasheet)				
Dose rate	Patient bodyweight (kg)	mg/kg range	No. of tablets required	
			57 mg	*227 mg*
Dogs				
5 mg/kg once daily	3–5.5	5.2–9.5	0.5	
	5.6–10	5.7–10.2	1	
	10.1–15	5.7–8.5	1.5	
	15.1–22	5.2–7.5		0.5
	22.1–45	5.0–10.3		1
	45.1–68	5.0–7.5		1.5
	68.1–90	5.0–6.7		2

Cats: *Do not use.*

Fluid volume loss calculations[4,8]

Non-acute fluid therapy

Clinical signs		Dehydration estimate (% of bodyweight)
Normal		<5%
Dry mucous membranes only		5%
Reduced skin turgor	Mild	6–8%
Increased heart rate	Moderate	8–10%
Weak pulses	Severe	10–12%
Collapse, shock		12–15%

Fluid deficit = % dehydration (see above table) x bodyweight x 10

Fluid maintenance requirements = 60 ml/kg/day for small dogs and cats; 40ml/kg/day for larger dogs

Daily fluid requirement = fluid deficit + maintenance requirement + ongoing losses (e.g. vomiting/diarrhoea)

Acute fluid therapy

Calculation of fluid volume needed:
1. Calculate the patient's normal blood volume (BV)
2. Estimate the percent blood loss, based on clinical signs and history
3. Calculate the volume deficit, VD = BV x % blood loss
4. Determine the resuscitation volume, based on:
   Whole blood volume = VD
   Colloid volume = 1.5 x VD
   Isotonic crystalloid volume = 4 x VD

Normal blood volume:	Dog = 80–90 ml/kg Cat = 60–70 ml/kg
Normal plasma volume:	Dog = 36–57 ml/kg Cat = 35–53 ml/kg

Shock fluid rates:

Isotonic crystalloid fluids Dog = 80–90 ml/kg/h Cat = 60–70 ml/kg/h	7.5% Hypertonic saline ± colloid 4 ml/kg over 10 minutes

Furosemide [16] (Frusemide)

(Dimazon, Frusecare, Frusedale, Frusol*) POM-V, POM

Formulations:

- Injectable: 50 mg/ml solution.
- Oral: 20 mg, 40 mg, 1 g tablets; 40 mg/5 ml oral solution.

DOSES

Dogs, Cats:

- Acute, life-threatening congestive heart failure: 1–4 mg/kg i.v., i.m. q1–4h as required, based on improvement in respiratory rate and effort. Once clinical signs improve, increase dosing interval to q8–12h, monitor urea, creatinine and electrolytes, and start oral therapy once tolerated.
- Chronic, congestive heart failure: 1–5 mg/kg p.o. q8–48h. Typical maintenance doses for mild to moderate CHF are 1–2 mg/kg p.o. q12–24h (dogs) and 1–2 mg/kg p.o. q12–48h (cats). The goal is to use the lowest dose of furosemide that effectively controls clinical signs. Doses in excess of 10 mg/kg/day (cats) or 15 mg/kg/day (dogs) are unlikely to be beneficial and additional diuretic therapy is required. In patients with ascites, use of s.c. instead of p.o. furosemide can have a marked clinical benefit.
- Hypercalciuric nephropathy: hydrate before therapy. Give 5 mg/kg bolus i.v., then begin 5 mg/kg/h infusion, or give 2–5 mg/kg i.v., s.c., p.o. q8–24h. Maintain hydration status and electrolyte balance with normal saline and added KCl. Furosemide generally reduces serum calcium levels by 0.5–1.5 mmol/l.
- Acute renal failure/uraemia: after replacing fluid deficit give furosemide at 2 mg/kg i.v. If no diuresis within 1 hour repeat dose at 4 mg/kg i.v. If no response within 1 hour give another dose at 6 mg/kg i.v. The use of low-dose dopamine as adjunctive therapy is often recommended.
- To promote diuresis in hyperkalaemic states: 2 mg/kg i.v. q6h.

Small mammals:

- Ferrets: 1–4 mg/kg i.v., i.m., p.o. q8–12h.
- Rabbits: 1–4 mg/kg i.v., i.m. q4–6h initially; maintenance doses are often 1–2 mg/kg p.o. q8–24h.
- Rodents: 1–4 mg/kg s.c., i.m. q4–6h or 5–10 mg/kg s.c., i.m. q12h.

Birds: 0.1–6.0 mg/kg i.m., s.c., i.v. q6–24h.

Reptiles: 5 mg/kg i.m. q12–24h.

NOTES

NOTES

NOTES

Gerbil biological data[14]

Lifespan (years)	2–3
Average weight (g) Males: Females:	 46–131 50–55
Number of digits Front: Rear:	 5 4
Heart rate (beats/min)	260–600
Respiratory rate (breaths/min)	85–160
Rectal temperature (°C)	37.4–39
Dentition	2 [I1/1 C0/0 P0/0 M3/3] Only incisors open-rooted
Environmental temperature (°C)	18–22
Relative humidity (%)	45–50
Daily water intake	4–5 ml
Fluid therapy	40–60 ml/kg/24h
Diet	Largely granivorous
Food intake per day per animal (g)	5–7
Coprophagy/Caecotrophy?	Yes
Oestrous type	Continuous polyoestrous
Post-partum oestrus?	Yes (resulting in delayed implantation)
Age at puberty (months)	Males: 2–4.5 Females: 2–3
Gestation length (days)	23–46
Oestrous cycle (days)	4–6
Oestrus duration (hours)	12–18
Litter size	3–8
Birth weight (g)	2.5–3.5
Altricial/Precocial	Altricial

Eyes open (days)	16–21
Age at weaning (days)	21–28
Number of pairs of teats	4
Minimum breeding age (months)	2.5–3.5
Ratio for breeding (M:F)	1:1 Form monogamous lifelong pairs in captivity. **Do not** remove the male
Comments	Pseudopregnancy is common following infertile mating, lasting 14–16 days

NOTES

Guinea pig biological data [14]

Lifespan (years)	5–6
Adult bodyweight (g)	Males: 900–1200 Females: 700–900
Dentition	2 [I 1/1, C0/0, P1/1, M3/3]
Body temperature (°C)	37.2–39.5
Heart rate (beats/min)	230–380
Respiratory rate (breaths/min)	90–150
Tidal volume (ml/kg)	5–10
Food consumption	6 g per 100 g bodyweight/day
Water consumption	10 ml per 100 g bodyweight/day
Sexual maturity (months)	Males: 3–4 (600–700 g) Females: 2–3 (350–450 g)
Oestrous cycle	15–17 days; breeding duration of 18–48 months
Duration of oestrus	1–16 hours
Gestation length (days)	59–72 (varies inversely with litter size, longer for small litters)
Parturition	Early morning. Farrowing: approximately 30 minutes; 5–10 minutes between pups
Post-partum oestrus	Yes
Litter size	1–6 (average 3–4)
Birth weight (g)	60–100; precocial; fully furred; ears open; teeth present
Eyes open (days)	Open at birth
Eat solid food (days)	May begin day after birth to nibble solid foods

NOTES

NOTES

NOTES

NOTES

Haemostasis – primary and secondary disorders[8]

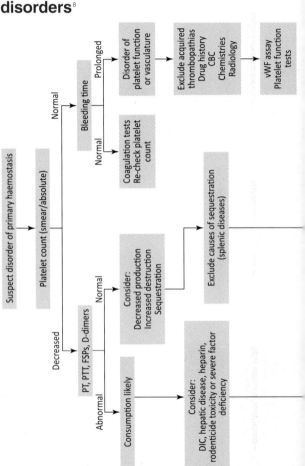

Suspect disorder of primary haemostasis

Platelet count (smear/absolute)

Normal

Bleeding time

- **Normal** → Coagulation tests / Re-check platelet count
- **Prolonged** → Disorder of platelet function or vasculature → Exclude acquired thrombopathias / Drug history / CBC / Chemistries / Radiology → vWF assay / Platelet function tests

Decreased

PT, PTT, FSPs, D-dimers

- **Normal** → Consider: Decreased production / Increased destruction / Sequestration → Exclude causes of sequestration (splenic diseases)
- **Abnormal** → Consumption likely → Consider: DIC, hepatic disease, heparin, rodenticide toxicity or severe factor deficiency

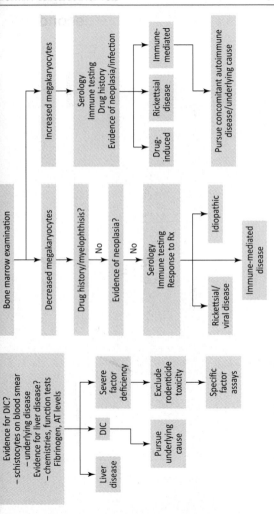

Approach to the diagnosis of disorders of primary haemostasis

AT = antithrombin; CBC = complete blood count; DIC = disseminated intravascular coagulation; FSPs = fibrin split products; PT = prothrombin time;
PTT = partial thromboplastin time; vWF = von Willebrand factor.

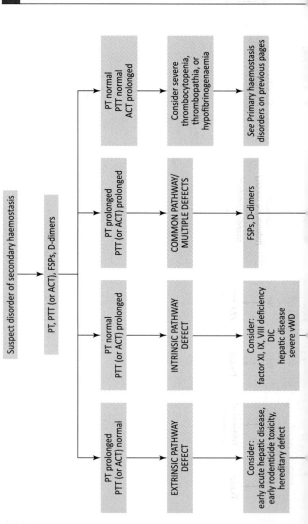

Suspect disorder of secondary haemostasis

↓

PT, PTT (or ACT), FSPs, D-dimers

PT prolonged / PTT (or ACT) normal
→ EXTRINSIC PATHWAY DEFECT
→ Consider: early acute hepatic disease, early rodenticide toxicity, hereditary defect

PT normal / PTT (or ACT) prolonged
→ INTRINSIC PATHWAY DEFECT
→ Consider: factor XI, IX, VIII deficiency, DIC, hepatic disease, severe vWD

PT prolonged / PTT (or ACT) prolonged
→ COMMON PATHWAY/ MULTIPLE DEFECTS
→ FSPs, D-dimers

PT normal / PTT normal / ACT prolonged
→ Consider severe thrombocytopenia, thrombopathia, or hypofibrinogenaemia
→ *See Primary haemostasis disorders on previous pages*

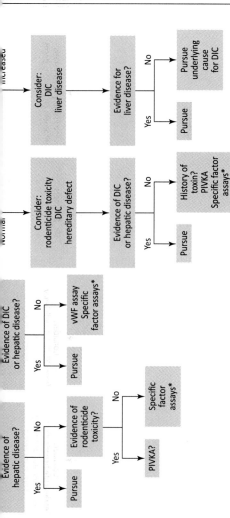

Approach to the diagnosis of disorders of secondary haemostasis

*See also Clotting factor tests.

ACT = activated coagulation time; DIC = disseminated intravascular coagulation; FSPs = fibrin split products; PIVKA = test for proteins induced by vitamin K absence/antagonism; PT = prothrombin time; PTT = partial thromboplastin time; vWF = von Willebrand factor; vWD = von Willebrand's disease.

Hamster biological data [14]

Lifespan (years)	1.5–2
Average weight (g) Males: Females:	 87–130 95–130
Number of digits Front: Rear:	 4 5
Heart rate (beats/min)	300–470
Respiratory rate (breaths/min)	40–110
Rectal temperature (°C)	36.2–37.5
Dentition	2 [I1/1 C0/0 P0/0 M3/3] Only incisors open-rooted
Environmental temperature (°C)	21–24
Relative humidity (%)	40–60
Daily water intake	10 ml/100g
Fluid therapy	100 ml/kg/24h
Diet	Omnivorous
Food intake per day per animal (g)	10–15
Coprophagy/Caecotrophy?	Yes
Oestrous type	Seasonal polyoestrous
Post-partum oestrus?	No
Age at puberty (months)	Males: 2 Females: 1.5
Gestation length (days)	Syrian: 16–18 Russian: 18–21 Chinese: 21–23 Roborovski: 23–30
Oestrous cycle (days)	4–5
Oestrus duration (hours)	8–26
Litter size	5–10
Birth weight (g)	1.5–3

Altricial/Precocial	Altricial
Eyes open (days)	12–14
Age at weaning (days)	19–21
Number of pairs of teats	6–7
Minimum breeding age (months)	2
Ratio for breeding (M:F)	1:1 Remove male after mating (except for Russian hamsters)
Comments	A vaginal discharge on day 2 of the oestrous cycle is normal and should not be confused with pyometra Cannibalism will occur if handled within 5 days of parturition Born with erupted incisors

NOTES

Head trauma – approach to management [11]

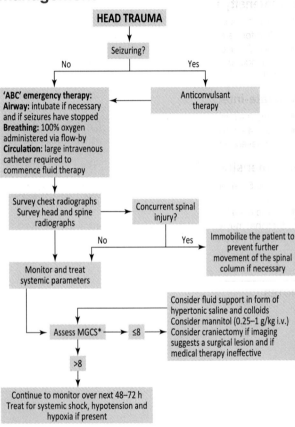

HEAD TRAUMA

Seizuring?

No — Yes

Yes → Anticonvulsant therapy

'ABC' emergency therapy:
Airway: intubate if necessary and if seizures have stopped
Breathing: 100% oxygen administered via flow-by
Circulation: large intravenous catheter required to commence fluid therapy

↓

Survey chest radiographs
Survey head and spine radiographs → Concurrent spinal injury?

No ↓   Yes → Immobilize the patient to prevent further movement of the spinal column if necessary

Monitor and treat systemic parameters

↓

Assess MGCS* — ≤8 → Consider fluid support in form of hypertonic saline and colloids
Consider mannitol (0.25–1 g/kg i.v.)
Consider craniectomy if imaging suggests a surgical lesion and if medical therapy ineffective

>8 ↓

Continue to monitor over next 48–72 h
Treat for systemic shock, hypotension and hypoxia if present

An approach to management of head trauma
*See Modified Glasgow Coma Scale (MGCS).

Heart murmur grading[5]

Low-intensity murmurs

- Grade 1 – a low-intensity murmur heard in a quiet environment only after careful auscultation over a localized cardiac area.
- Grade 2 – a low-intensity murmur heard immediately when the stethoscope is placed over the point of maximum intensity (PMI).

Moderate-intensity murmurs

- Grade 3 – a murmur of moderate intensity.
- Grade 4 – a high-intensity murmur that can be auscultated over several areas without any palpable precordial thrill.

High-intensity murmurs

- Grade 5 – a high-intensity murmur with a palpable precordial thrill.
- Grade 6 – a high-intensity murmur with a palpable precordial thrill that may even be heard when the stethoscope is slightly lifted off the chest wall.

NOTES

Heart radiograph – 'clock face' analogy[5]

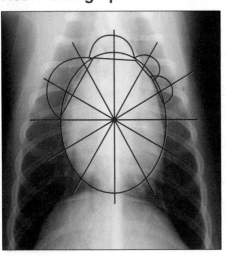

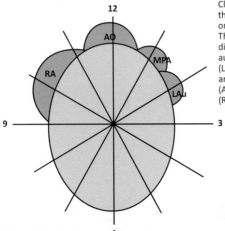

Clock face analogy of the cardiac silhouette on a DV or VD view. The location of dilatation of the left auricular appendage (LAu), main pulmonary artery (MPA), aorta (AO) and right atrium (RA) are shown.

Heart – vertebral heart score[13]

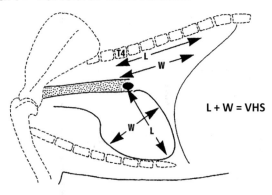

Technique to perform a VHS on a lateral radiograph

L = Length of the cardiac silhouette; T4 = Fourth thoracic vertebra; W = Width of the cardiac silhouette. Reproduced from Dennis R *et al.* (2001) *Handbook of Small Animal Radiological Differential Diagnosis*, p.126. © Elsevier)

Normal vertebral heart score

v = vertebrae

Dog mean value

9.7 ± 0.5

Dog breed-specific values

Boxer: 11.6 ± 0.8 v
Cavalier King Charles Spaniel: 10.6 ± 0.5 v
Dobermann: 10.0 ± 0.6 v
German Shepherd Dog: 9.7 ± 0.7 v
Labrador Retriever: 10.8 ± 0.6 v
Whippet: 11.0 ± 0.5 v
Yorkshire Terrier: 9.7 ± 0.5 v

Puppies

Have VHS values within the same 8.5–10.5 v range

Cats

7.5 ± 0.3 v on a lateral view
(The cardiac width on a DV/VD view is 3.4 ± 0.25 v if measured perpendicular to the long axis)

Hypertension [19]

Risk category	Systolic blood pressure (mmHg)	Recommendation for starting treatment
Minimal	<150	■ Minimal to mild risk of developing target organ damage (TOD) ■ Limited evidence that anti-hypertensive medication required ■ May represent cases of 'white-coat' hypertension ■ Treatment should be considered if evidence of ocular or central nervous system TOD ■ Continued monitoring recommended ■ Target categories for patients treated with anti-hypertensive therapies
Mild	150–159	
Moderate	160–179	■ Moderate risk for the development of TOD ■ Anti-hypertensive therapy recommended in patients with evidence of TOD or where concurrent clinical conditions associated with hypertension have been identified ■ Confirmation of hypertensive category status should be made on at least two occasions unless there is evidence of ocular or CNS TOD, when therapy will be required immediately ■ Patients in this category which have no evidence of TOD or clinical conditions associated with systemic hypertension should be monitored carefully to exclude white-coat hypertension before a diagnosis of idiopathic hypertension is made and long-term treatment started
Severe	>180	■ The risk of development and progression of TOD is high ■ White-coat hypertension is uncommon ■ Immediate anti-hypertensive therapy indicated if ocular or CNS TOD present otherwise confirmation of category status should be made on at least two occasions

ACVIM risk categories for systolic hypertension in dogs and cats

NOTES

NOTES

NOTES

NOTES

Imidacloprid [16]

(Advantage, Advantix, Advocate, Bob Martin Double Action
Dewormer) POM-V, AVM-GSL

Formulations:

- Topical: 100 mg/ml imidacloprid in spot-on pipettes of various
  sizes (Advantage, Bob Martin).
- Topical for cat: 100 mg/ml imidacloprid with moxidectin in
  spot-on pipette (Advocate).
- Topical for dog: 100 mg/ml imidacloprid + 500 mg/ml
  permethrin in spot-on pipettes of various sizes (Advantix);
  100 mg/ml imidacloprid with moxidectin in spot-on pipette
  (Advocate).

DOSES

Dogs: 0.4 ml, 1.0 ml, 2.5 ml, 4 ml pipettes. In dogs >40 kg the
appropriate combination of pipettes should be applied.

Cats: 0.4 ml, 0.8 ml pipettes (use the smaller size in cats <4 kg).
Do not use the permethrin-containing product.

Small mammals:

- Ferrets: 0.4 ml pipette q30d.
- Rabbits 0.4 ml, 0.8 ml pipettes (use the smaller size in rabbits
  <4 kg).

NOTES

Insulin [16]

(Caninsulin, Actrapid*, Humulin*, Hypurin*, Insulatard*, Lantus*)
POM-V, POM

Formulations: Injectable: 40 IU/ml, 100 IU/ml suspensions (for s.c. injection) or 100 IU/ml solution (for s.c., i.v. or i.m. injection). There are many preparations (including lente and PZI) authorized for use in humans; however, veterinary authorized preparations, when available, are preferential for both legal and medical reasons.

Route	Onset	Peak effect in dog (hours)	Peak effect in cat (hours)	Duration of action in dog (hours)	Duration of action in cat (hours)
Soluble (neutral)					
i.v.	Immediate	0.5–2	0.5–2	1–4	1–4
i.m.	10–30 min	1–4	1–4	3–8	3–8
s.c.	10–30 min	1–5	1–5	4–8	4–8
Semilente (amorphous IZS)					
s.c.	30–60 min	1–5	1–5	4–10	4–10
Isophane (NPH)					
s.c.	0.5–3 h	2–10	2–8	6–24	4–12
Lente (mixed IZS)					
s.c.	30–60 min	2–10	2–8	8–24	6–14
Ultralente (crystalline IZS)					
s.c.	2–8 h	4–16	4–16	8–28	8–24
PZI					
s.c.	1–4 h	4–14	3–12	6–28	6–24
Glargine					
s.c.	1–4 h	Unknown	3–12	Unknown	12–24

IZS = Insulin zinc suspension; NPH = Neutral protamine Hagedorn; PZI = Protamine zinc insulin.
Note that all times are approximate averages and insulin doses need to be adjusted for individual patients.

Trade name	Species of insulin	Types available
Actrapid*	Human	Neutral
Caninsulin	Porcine	Lente
Lantus*	Human	Glargine
Humulin*	Human	Neutral, Isophane
Hypurin*	Bovine	Neutral, Isophane, Lente, PZI
	Porcine	Neutral, Isophane
Insulatard*	Human or porcine	Isophane

* = Not authorized for veterinary use.

DOSES

Dogs:

- Insulin-dependent diabetes mellitus: Initially 0.25–0.5 IU/kg (dogs >25 kg) or 0.5–1 IU/kg (dogs <25 kg) of lente insulin s.c. q12–24h. Adjust dose and frequency of administration by monitoring clinical effect, urine results, blood glucose and/or fructosamines.
- Diabetic ketoacidosis: 0.2 IU/kg soluble insulin i.m. initially followed by 0.1 IU/kg i.m. q1h. Alternatively i.v. infusions may be given (though are not reported to be better) at 0.025–0.06 IU/kg/h of soluble insulin. Run approximately 50 ml of i.v. solution through tubing as insulin adheres to glass and plastic; change insulin/saline solution q6h.
- Hyperkalaemic myocardial toxicity (not in hypoadrenocorticism): give a bolus of 0.5 IU/kg of soluble insulin i.v. followed by 2–3 g of dextrose/unit of insulin. Half the dextrose should be given as a bolus and the remainder administered i.v. over 4–6h.

Cats:

- Insulin-dependent diabetes mellitus: Initially 0.25 IU/kg of lente insulin s.c. q12h or 0.25 IU/kg of glargine insulin (or PZI if available) s.c. q12–24h. Adjust dose and frequency of administration by monitoring clinical effect, urine results, blood glucose and/or fructosamine levels.
- Diabetic ketoacidosis: Doses as for dogs.
- Hyperkalaemic myocardial toxicity: Doses as for dogs. ➡

Small mammals: Ferrets: Lente insulin 0.5–1.0 IU/ferret q12h.

Reptiles:

- Chelonians, Snakes: 1–5 IU/kg i.m. q24–72h.
- Crocodilians, Lizards: 5–10 IU/kg i.m. q24–72h; adjust doses according to serial glucose measurement.

Intraocular pressure (IOP) normal values

- **Dogs:** 10–25 mmHg [17]
- **Most other species:** 15–25 mmHg; the difference between fellow eyes should be less than 8 mmHg [18]

Ivermectin [16]

(Alstomec, Animec, Bimectin, Ivomec, Panomec, Qualimintic, Virbamec, Xeno 450, Xeno 50-mini,) POM-V, POM-VPS, SAES

Formulations:

- Injectable: 1% w/v solution.
- Topical: 100 µg/g, 800 µg/g spot-on tubes; 200 µg/ml spray (Xeno).

DOSES

Dogs:

- Sarcoptic mange: 200–400 µg (micrograms)/kg p.o., s.c. q2w for 4–6 weeks.
- Cheyletiellosis: 200–300 µg (micrograms)/kg p.o., s.c. q1–2w for 6–8 weeks.
- Generalized demodicosis: 300–600 µg (micrograms)/kg p.o., s.c. daily.

Cats: Otoacariasis (*Otodectes cynotis* infestation): 1% w/v ivermection diluted 1:9 with propylene glycol topically (in affected ears) 1 drop daily for 21 days.

Small mammals: 0.2–0.5 mg/kg s.c., p.o. q7–14d.

- Ferrets, Rabbits, Guinea pigs: apply 450 µg (micrograms)/kg (1 tube Xeno 450) topically.
- Ferrets, small rodents <800 g: 50 µg (micrograms)/250g (15 drops Xeno 50-mini) q7–14d.

Birds: 200 µg (micrograms)/kg i.m., s.c., p.o. q7–14d.
- Raptors: capillariasis: 0.5–1 mg/kg i.m., p.o. q7–14d; *Serratospiculum*: 1 mg/kg p.o., i.m. q7–14d (moxidectin or doramectin may be given at same dose rates).
- Passerines and small psittacids: systemic dosing as above or 0.2 mg/kg applied topically to skin using 0.02% solution (in propylene glycol) q7–14d.
- Pigeons: 0.5 ml applied topically to bare skin using 0.02% solution q7–14d.

Reptiles: 0.2 mg/kg s.c., p.o. once, repeat in 10–14 days until negative for parasites; may use as environmental control for snake mites (*Ophionyssus natricis*) at dilution of 5 mg/l water sprayed in tank q7–10d (if pre-mix ivermectin with propylene glycol this facilitates mixing with water)
- Chelonians: *do not use*.

NOTES

NOTES

NOTES

NOTES

Ketamine [16]

(Ketaset injection, Narketan-10, Vetalar-V) POM-V CD Schedule 4

Formulations: Injectable: 100 mg/ml solution.

DOSES

See **Sedation combinations** *for sedation protocols in all species.*

Dogs:
- Perioperative analgesia: Intraoperatively: 10 μg (micrograms)/kg/min, postoperatively: 2–5 μg (micrograms)/kg/min, both preceded by a 250 μg (micrograms)/kg loading dose. There is some evidence to suggest that a 10 μg/kg/min dose may be too low to provide adequate analgesia continuously, although other evidence-based dose recommendations are lacking.
- Induction of anaesthesia (combined with diazepam or midazolam) as part of a volatile anaesthetic technique: 2 mg/kg i.v.
- Induction of general anaesthesia combined with medetomidine or dexmedetomidine to provide a total injectable combination: ketamine (5–7 mg/kg i.m.) combined with medetomidine (40 μg (micrograms)/kg i.m.) or dexmedetomidine (20 μg (micrograms)/kg i.m.).

Cats:
- Chemical restraint: ketamine (5 mg/kg i.m.) combined with midazolam or diazepam (0.2 mg/kg i.m.), reduce dose of ketamine to 2.5 mg/kg if using i.v.; increasing the dose of ketamine (10 mg/kg i.m.) if combined with a benzodiazepine (as above) will provide a short period of general anaesthesia.
- Combinations of ketamine (5–7.5 mg/kg i.m.) combined with medetomidine (80 μg (micrograms)/kg i.m.) or dexmedetomidine (40 μg (micrograms)/kg i.m.) will provide 20–30 min general anaesthesia. Reduce the doses of both drugs when given i.v.
- Doses for provision of perioperative analgesia are the same as those for dogs.

Small mammals:

- Ferrets: 10–30 mg/kg i.m., s.c. alone gives immobilization and some analgesia but may have prolonged recovery at this high dose. For general anaesthesia, sedate first and then induce with isoflurane; alternatively, combinations of ketamine (5–8 mg/kg) with medetomidine (0.08–0.1 mg/kg i.m., s.c.) or dexmedetomidine (0.04–0.05 mg/kg i.m., s.c.) will provide 20 minutes of general anaesthesia.

- Rabbits: 15–30 mg/kg i.m., s.c. alone gives moderate to heavy sedation with some analgesia but may have long recovery at this high dose.

- Guinea pigs: 10–50 mg/kg i.m., s.c. will provide immobilization, with little muscle relaxation and some analgesia, however it is suggested to use the lower end of the dose range to sedate first and then induce with isoflurane; alternatively, a combination of ketamine (4–5 mg/kg i.m., s.c.) with medetomidine (0.05 mg/kg i.m., s.c.) or dexmedetomidine (0.025 mg/kg i.m., s.c.) will provide a short period of anaesthesia.

- Other rodents: 10–50 mg/kg i.m., s.c. will provide immobilization, however it is suggested to use the lower end of the dose range and to induce anaesthesia with isoflurane.

Birds: Largely superseded by gaseous anaesthesia.

Reptiles:

- Chelonians: 20–60 mg/kg i.m., i.v.
- Lizards: 25–60 mg/kg i.m., i.v.
- Snakes: 20–80 mg/kg i.m., i.v.

NOTES

NOTES

Lactulose [16]
(Lactugal*, Lactulose*) P

Formulations: Oral: 3.1–3.7 g/5 ml lactulose in a syrup base.

DOSES

Dogs:
- Constipation: 5–25 ml p.o. q8h. Monitor and adjust therapy to produce two or three soft stools per day.
- Acute hepatic encephalopathy: 18–20 ml/kg of a solution comprising 3 parts lactulose to 7 parts water per rectum as a retention enema for 4–8h. Monitor and adjust therapy to produce two or three soft stools per day.

Cats: 0.5–5 ml p.o. q8–12h.

Ferrets: 0.15–0.75 ml/kg p.o. q12h.

Birds: Appetite stimulant, hepatic encephalopathy: 0.2–1 ml/kg p.o. q8–12h.

Reptiles: 0.5 ml/kg p.o. q24h.

NOTES

Levothyroxine [16] (T4, L-Thyroxine)
(Forthyron, Leventa, Soloxine, Thyroxyl) POM-V

Formulations: Oral: 0.1 mg, 0.2 mg, 0.3 mg, 0.5 mg, 0.8 mg tablets; 1 mg/ml solution.

DOSES

Dogs, Cats: 0.02–0.04 mg/kg/day. Alternatively dose at 0.5 mg/m^2 body surface area daily (see Bodyweight to body surface area conversion tables). Dose once or divided twice a day according to response. Monitor serum T4 levels pre-dosing and 4–8 hours after dosing.

Leventa (from datasheet)					
Dose rate	Patient bodyweight (kg)	Volume required (ml)			
		Dosage 10 µg/kg	Dosage 20 µg/kg	Dosage 30 µg/kg	Dosage 40 µg/kg
Dogs					
Recommended starting dose of 20 µg/kg once daily	5	0.05	0.10	0.15	0.20
	10	0.10	0.20	0.30	0.40
	15	0.15	0.30	0.45	0.60
	20	0.20	0.40	0.60	0.80
	25	0.25	0.50	0.75	1.00
	30	0.30	0.60	0.90	1.20
	35	0.35	0.70	1.05	1.40
	40	0.40	0.80	1.20	1.60
	45	0.45	0.90	1.35	1.80
	50	0.50	1.00	1.50	2.00

Birds: 0.02 mg/kg p.o. q12–24h. Dissolve 1 mg in 28.4 ml water and give 0.4–0.5 ml/kg q12–24h.

Reptiles: Tortoises: 0.02 mg/kg p.o. q24–48h.

Lufenuron [16]

(Program, Program Plus) POM-V

Formulations:
- Oral: 67.8 mg, 204.9 mg, 409.8 mg tablets (Program); 46 mg, 115 mg, 230 mg, 460 mg lufeneron with milbemycin (ratio of 20 mg lufeneron: 1 mg milbemycin) tablets (Program Plus); 133 mg, 266 mg suspension (Program for cats).
- Injectable: 40 mg, 80 mg as 100 mg/ml suspension (Program).

DOSES

Dogs: 10 mg/kg p.o., s.c. q1month (equivalent to a dose of 0.5 mg/kg milbemycin in combined preparations).

Cats: 10 mg/kg s.c. q6months or 30 mg/kg p.o. q1month.

Ferrets: 30–45 mg/kg p.o. q1month.

NOTES

NOTES

NOTES

NOTES

Maropitant [16]

(Cerenia) POM-V

Formulations:

- Injectable: 10 mg/ml solution.
- Oral: 16 mg, 24 mg, 60 mg, 160 mg tablets.

DOSES

Dogs: 1 mg/kg s.c. q24h or 2 mg/kg p.o. q24h. For prevention of motion sickness, tablets at a dose rate of 8 mg/kg q24h for a maximum of 2 days are indicated.

Cerenia (from datasheet)					
Dose rate	**Patient bodyweight (kg)**	**No. of tablets required**			
		16 mg	*24 mg*	*60 mg*	*160 mg*
Dogs					
Treatment and prevention of vomiting (except motion sickness): 2 mg/kg once daily *(Not to be used in dogs <8 weeks old)*	3.0–4.0*	½			
	4.1–8.0	1			
	8.1–12.0		1		
	12.1–24.0		2		
	24.1–30.0			1	
	30.1–60.0			2	
Prevention of motion sickness only: 8 mg/kg once daily *(Not to be used in dogs <16 weeks old)*	1.0–1.5		½		
	1.6–2.0	1			
	2.1–3.0		1		
	3.1–4.0	2			
	4.1–6.0		2		
	6.1–7.5			1	
	7.6–10.0				½
	10.1–15.0			2	
	15.1–20.0				1
	20.1–30.0				1½
	30.1–40.0				2
	40.1–60.0				3

Correct dose for dogs <3 kg cannot be accurately achieved.

➡

Cats: Not authorized. However, 0.5–1 mg/kg p.o., s.c. q24h is likely to be effective in reducing emesis from 2 to 24 hours after dosing. Tolerance has been demonstrated at 5 mg/kg s.c. q24h for a maximum of 15 days.

Medetomidine [16]

(Domitor, Dorbene, Dormilan, Medetor, Sedastart, Sedator, Sededorm) POM-V

Formulations: Injectable: 1 mg/ml solution.

DOSES

Dogs, Cats: Premedication: 10–20 µg (micrograms)/kg i.v., i.m, s.c in combination with an opioid. Use lower end of dose range i.v.

Small mammals: Premedication: 80–100 µg (micrograms) i.m., s.c. in combination with an opioid and ketamine.

Reptiles: 100–200 µg (micrograms)/kg i.m; may be combined with 5–10 mg/kg ketamine to provide light anaesthesia.

See also **Premedication protocols – drug combinations used in dogs and cats *and* Sedation combinations**

Meloxicam [16]

(Actiam, Adocam, Flexicam, Loxicam, Melovem, Meloxidyl, Meloxivet, Metacam, Rheumocam) POM-V

Formulations:
- Oral: 0.5 mg/ml suspension for cats, 1.5 mg/ml oral suspension for dogs; 1.0 mg, 2.5 mg tablets for dogs.
- Injectable: 2 mg/ml solution for cats, 5 mg/ml solution.

DOSES

Dogs: Initial dose is 0.2 mg/kg s.c., p.o.; if given as a single preoperative injection effects last for 24 hours. Can be followed by a maintenance dose of 0.1 mg/kg p.o q24h.

Metacam Chewable Tablets for Dogs (from datasheet)				
Dose rate	Patient bodyweight (kg)	No. of tablets per dose, once daily		mg/kg
		1 mg	2.5 mg	
Dogs				
0.1 mg/kg (maintenance dose)	4.0–7.0	½		0.13–0.1
	7.1–10.0	1		0.14–0.1
	10.1–15.0	1½		0.15–0.1
	15.1–20.0	2		0.13–0.1
	20.1–25.0		1	0.12–0.1
	25.1–35.0		1½	0.15–0.1
	35.1–50.0		2	0.14–0.1

Cats:

- Initial injectable dose is 0.2 mg/kg s.c.; if given as a single preoperative injection effects last for 24 hours. To continue treatment for up to 5 days, may be followed 24 h later by the oral suspension for cats at a dosage of 0.05 mg/kg p.o.
- Postoperative pain/inflammation: single injection of 0.3 mg/kg s.c. has been shown to be safe and efficacious. It is *not* recommended to follow this with oral meloxicam 24 hours later.
- Chronic pain: initial oral dose is 0.1 mg/kg p.o. q24h, which can be followed by a maintenance dose of 0.05 mg/kg p.o q24h. Treatment should be discontinued after 14 days if no clinical improvement is apparent.

Small mammals:

- Rabbits: 0.3–0.6 mg/kg s.c., p.o. q24h; studies have shown that rabbits may require a dose exceeding 0.3 mg/kg q24h to achieve optimal plasma levels of meloxicam over a 24-hour interval and doses of 1.5 mg/kg s.c., p.o. are well tolerated for 5 days.
- Rats: 1–2 mg/kg s.c., p.o. q24h.
- Mice: 2 mg/kg s.c. p.o. q24h.

Birds: 0.5–1.0 mg/kg i.m., p.o. q12–24h.

Reptiles: 0.2 mg/kg i.m., p.o. q24h.

Metaflumizone [16]

(Promeris, Promeris Duo) POM-V

Formulations: Topical: 200 mg/ml spot-on pipettes of various sizes (Promeris); 150 mg/ml metaflumizone + 150 mg/ml amitraz in various sizes (Promeris Duo).

DOSES

Dogs, Cats: 40 mg/kg applied topically every 4–6 weeks. *Do not use Promeris Duo in cats.*

Methimazole [16]

(Felimazole) POM-V

Formulations: Oral: 2.5 mg, 5 mg tablet.

DOSES

Dogs: 2.5–5 mg/dog p.o. q12h depending on size.

Cats: 2.5 mg/cat p.o. q12h.

Reptiles: Snakes: 2 mg/kg p.o. q24h for 30 days.

Methoprene [16] (S-Methoprene)

(Acclaim spray, Frontline Combo, R.I.P fleas) NFA-VPS, GSL

Formulations:
- Topical: 10% w/v fipronil with *S*-methoprene in spot-on pipettes of various sizes (Frontline).
- Environmental: *S*-methoprene + permethrin household spray (Acclaim); *S*-methoprene, tetramethrin + permethrin household spray (R.I.P Fleas).

DOSES

Dogs, Cats: 1 pipette per animal monthly according to body weight. Cheyletiellosis, Otoacariasis (*Otodectes cynotis* infestation): two applications 4 weeks apart.

Rabbits: *Do not use.*

Birds: *Do not use.*

Metronidazole [16]

Metronidazole, Stomorgyl, Flagyl*, Metrolyl*) POM-V, POM

Formulations:

- Injectable: 5 mg/ml i.v. infusion.
- Oral: 200 mg, 400 mg, 500 mg tablets; 25 mg metronidazole + 46.9 mg spiramycin tablets, 125 mg metronidazole + 234.4 mg spiramycin tablets, 250 mg metronidazole + 469 mg spiramycin tablets (Stomorgyl); 40 mg/ml oral solution.

DOSES

Dogs:

- Flagyl: 15–25 mg/kg p.o. q12h or 10 mg/kg s.c., slow i.v. infusion q12h. Use higher doses, 25 mg/kg p.o. q12h, for protozoal infections. Injectable solution may be given intrapleurally to treat empyema.
- Stomorgyl: 12.5 mg metronidazole + 23.4 mg spiramycin/kg p.o. q24h for 5–10 days.

Cats:

- 8–10 mg/kg i.v., p.o. q12h. Injectable solution may be given intrapleurally to treat empyema.
- Stomorgyl: 12.5 mg metronidazole + 23.4 mg spiramycin/kg p.o. q24h for 5–10 days.

Stomorgyl Film-coated Tablets (from datasheet)			
Dose rate	No. of tablets per dose, once daily		
	STOMORGYL 2 (most suitable for use in cats)	STOMORGYL 10	STOMORGYL 20
Dogs and cats			
23.4 mg spiramycin and 12.5 mg metronidazole/ kg once daily for 5 to 10 days	1 per 2 kg bodyweight	1 per 10 kg bodyweight	1 per 20 kg bodyweight

→

Small mammals:

- Ferrets: 15–20 mg/kg p.o q12h; 50–75 mg/kg p.o. q24h for 14 days with clarithromycin and omeprazole for *Helicobacter*.
- Rabbits, Chinchillas, Guinea pigs: 10–20 mg/kg p.o. q12h, 40 mg/kg p.o. q24h; 50 mg/kg p.o. q12h for 5 days may be required for giardiasis in chinchillas but use with caution.
- Rats, Mice: 20 mg/kg s.c. q24h.
- Other rodents: 20–40 mg/kg p.o. q24h.

Birds:

- Raptors: 50 mg/kg p.o. q24h for 5 days.
- Pigeons: 40–50 mg/kg p.o. q24h for 5–7 days or 100 mg/kg p.o. q48h for 3 doses or 200 mg/kg p.o. once.
- Parrots: 30 mg/kg p.o. q12h.
- Passerines: 50 mg/kg p.o. q12h or 200 mg/l water daily for 7 days.

Reptiles:

- Anaerobic bacterial infections: Iguanas, Snakes: 20 mg/kg p.o q24–48h.
- Protozoal infections: Indigo Snake, Kingsnake, Milksnakes: 40 mg/kg p.o., repeat after 14 days; Other snakes: 100 mg/kg p.o., repeat after 14 days; Chelonians: 100–125 mg/kg p.o., repeat after 14 days (use lower doses of 50 mg/kg p.o. q24h for 3–5 days for severe infections); Chameleons: 40–60 mg/kg p.o., repeat after 14 days.

MGCS *see* **Modified Glasgow Coma Scale**

NOTES

Milbemycin [16]

Milbemax, Program Plus) POM-V

Formulations: Oral: 2.5 mg/25 mg, 12.5 mg/125 mg milbemycin/
praziquantel tablets (Milbemax for dogs); 4 mg/10 mg, 16 mg/40 mg
Milbemax for cats); 2.3 mg, 5.75 mg, 11.5 mg, 23 mg milbemycin
with lufenuron (ratio 20 mg lufeneron: 1 mg milbemycin) tablets
Program Plus).

DOSES

Dogs:
- With lufenuron: 0.5 mg milbemycin/kg + 10 mg lufeneron/kg
  p.o. q30d.
- With praziquantel: 0.5 mg/kg milbemycin + 5 mg/kg
  praziquantel p.o. q30d. For *Angiostrongylus vasorum*:
  administer same dose 4 times at weekly intervals.

Cats: 2 mg/kg milbemycin + 5 mg/kg praziquantel p.o. q30d.

Milbemax (from datasheet)			
Dose rate	Patient bodyweight (kg)	No. of tablets required	
		MILBEMAX tablets for small dogs and puppies/small cats and kittens, respectively	*MILBEMAX tablets for dogs/cats, respectively*
Dogs			
0.5 mg milbemycin oxime and 5 mg praziquantel per kg	1–5 kg	1	
	5–25 kg		1
	>25–50 kg		2
	>50–75 kg		3
Cats			
2 mg milbemycin oxime and 5 mg praziquantel per kg	0.5–1 kg	½	
	>1–2 kg	1	
	>2–4 kg		½
	>4–8 kg		1
	>8–12 kg		1 ½

Ferrets: 1.15–2.33 mg/kg p.o. q30d.

Reptiles: Chelonians: 0.25–0.5 mg/kg s.c.

Modified Glasgow Coma Scale (MGCS)[8]

Motor activity	Score
Normal gait, normal spinal reflexes	6
Hemiparesis, tetraparesis or decerebrate rigidity	5
Recumbent, intermittent extensor rigidity	4
Recumbent, constant extensor rigidity	3
Recumbent, constant extensor rigidity with opisthotonus	2
Recumbent, hypotonia of muscles, depressed or absent spinal reflexes	1
Brainstem reflexes	
Normal pupillary light reflexes and oculocephalic reflexes	6
Slow pupillary light reflexes and normal to reduced oculocephalic reflexes	5
Bilateral unresponsive miosis with normal to reduced oculocephalic reflexes	4
Pinpoint pupils with reduced to absent oculocephalic reflexes	3
Unilateral, unresponsive mydriasis with reduced to absent oculocephalic reflexes	2
Bilateral, unresponsive mydriasis with reduced to absent oculocephalic reflexes	1
Level of consciousness	
Occasional periods of alertness and responsive to environment	6
Depression or delirium, capable of responding but response may be inappropriate	5
Semi-comatose, responsive to visual stimuli	4
Semi-comatose, responsive to auditory stimuli	3
Semi-comatose, responsive only to repeated noxious stimuli	2
Comatose, unresponsive to repeated noxious stimuli	1

This provides a total score of 3 to 18. The higher the score, the better the prognosis.

Mouse biological data [14]

Lifespan (years)	1–2.5
Average weight (g) Males: Females:	 20–40 20–60
Number of digits Front: Rear:	 4 5
Heart rate (beats/min)	420–700
Respiratory rate (breaths/min)	100–250
Rectal temperature (°C)	~37.5
Dentition	2 [I1/1 C0/0 P0/0 M3/3] Only incisors open-rooted
Environmental temperature (°C)	24–25
Relative humidity (%)	45–55
Daily water intake	15 ml/100 g
Fluid therapy	100 ml/kg/24h
Diet	Omnivorous
Food intake per day per animal (g)	3–5
Coprophagy/Caecotrophy?	Yes
Oestrous type	Continuous polyoestrous
Post-partum oestrus?	Yes
Age at puberty (months)	1.5
Gestation length (days)	19–21
Oestrous cycle (days)	4–5
Oestrus duration (hours)	9–20
Litter size	7–12
Birth weight (g)	1–1.5
Altricial/Precocial	Altricial

Eyes open (days)	12–14
Age at weaning (days)	18–21
Number of pairs of teats	5
Minimum breeding age (months)	2
Ratio for breeding (M:F)	1:1–6 If polygamous remove female before parturition
Comments	They will eat the litter if disturbed in the first 2–3 days

Moxidectin [16]

(Advocate) POM-V

Formulations:

- Topical for cat: 10 mg/ml moxidectin with imidacloprid in spot-on pipette.
- Topical for dog: 25 mg/ml moxidectin with imidacloprid in spot-on pipette.

DOSES

Dogs: 0.4 ml, 1.0 ml, 2.5 ml, 4 ml pipette according to size of dog. Apply once every month. Minimum dose recommendation 0.1 ml/kg.

Cats: 0.4 ml, 0.8 ml pipette according to size of cat. Apply once every month. Minimum dose recommendation 0.1 ml/kg.

Small mammals:
- Ferrets: 0.4 ml pipette monthly. If under heavy flea pressure can repeat once after 2 weeks.
- Rabbits: 0.2 mg/kg p.o., repeat in 10 days.
- Rodents: GI nematodes: 1 mg/kg of 2.5% v/w solution once.

Birds: 0.2 mg/kg topically prn.

NOTES

NOTES

NOTES

Neck pain – clinical approach [11]

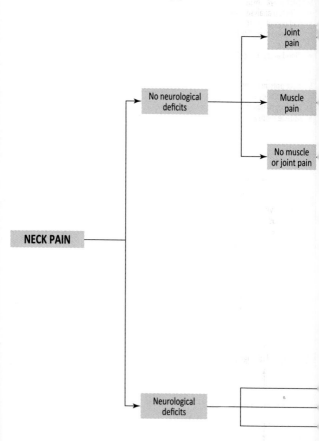

Clinical approach to neck pain

ANA = anti-nuclear antibody; CK =creatine kinase; CSF = cerebrospinal fluid; LE = lupus erythematosus; RhF = rheumatoid factor.

Suspect polyarthritis
- Joint tap analysis and culture
- Radiograph joints
- Antibody titres for infectious disease
- Blood and urine culture
- Serum LE, ANA, RhF
- Joint capsule biopsy
- Echocardiography
- Rule out intestinal disease
- Rule out systemic cancer

Suspect polymyositis
- Serum CK levels
- Electrophysiology
- Muscle biopsy
- Antibody titres for infectious disease
- Serum LE, ANA, RhF

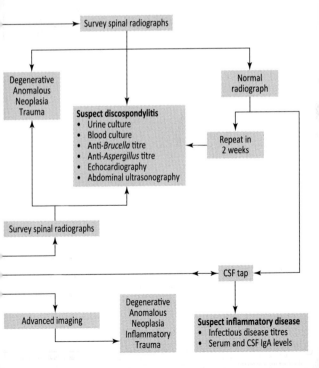

Survey spinal radiographs

Degenerative
Anomalous
Neoplasia
Trauma

Normal radiograph

Suspect discospondylitis
- Urine culture
- Blood culture
- Anti-*Brucella* titre
- Anti-*Aspergillus* titre
- Echocardiography
- Abdominal ultrasonography

Repeat in 2 weeks

Survey spinal radiographs

CSF tap

Advanced imaging

Degenerative
Anomalous
Neoplasia
Inflammatory
Trauma

Suspect inflammatory disease
- Infectious disease titres
- Serum and CSF IgA levels

NOTES

NOTES

NOTES

Ortolani test[3]

Indications/Use

- To detect hip laxity in the young dog (to support a diagnosis of hip dysplasia)

> Not all dogs with hip dysplasia show a positive Ortolani sign. For example, dogs with gross subluxation or luxation of the femoral head, and dogs in which capsular fibrosis has stabilized the hip joint will not show the sign.

Patient preparation and positioning

- May be attempted in the conscious animal but is potentially painful and therefore best performed with the dog heavily sedated or under general anaesthesia.
- The animal may be positioned in lateral or dorsal recumbency. The description below applies to lateral recumbency.

Technique

1. Position the stifle in mild flexion and grasp it with one hand, with the other hand placed on the dorsal aspect of the pelvis to stabilize it.
2. Apply firm pressure to the stifle in a dorsal direction in an attempt to subluxate the hip joint.
3. Whilst maintaining dorsal pressure on the stifle, gently abduct the limb until a 'click' or 'clunk' is detected.
   - If the dorsal acetabular rim is intact, the femoral head falls abruptly into the acetabulum.

(ii) Abduction

(i) Dorsal pressure

➡

- In dogs with a poor dorsal acetabular rim, the femoral head appears to slide back into the acetabulum.
4. Whilst maintaining dorsal pressure on the stifle, if the limb is now adducted, re-luxation of the hip will occur.

Results

- The 'click' or 'clunk' (see Step 3) represents the relocation of the femoral head within the acetabulum. This is the positive Ortolani sign, consistent with hip joint laxity.

NOTES

Otitis externa/media – clinical approach[7]

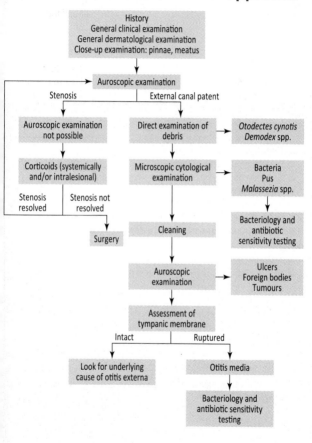

A practical approach to otitis externa and otitis media

Adapted from DN Carlotti

Oxytetracycline [16]
(Engemycin, Oxycare) POM-V

Formulations:

- Injectable: 50 mg/ml solution.
- Oral: 50 mg, 100 mg, 250 mg tablets. Feed supplement and soluble powders also available.

DOSES

Dogs: 7–11 mg/kg i.m., s.c. q24h; 10–20 mg/kg p.o. q8h. Give oral dose on an empty stomach.

Cats: 7–11 mg/kg i.m., s.c. q24h.

Small mammals:

- Ferrets, Hamsters, Gerbils: 20–25 mg/kg i.m. q8–12h.
- Rabbits: 15 mg/kg i.m. q12h.
- Chinchillas: 15 mg/kg i.m. q12h; 50 mg/kg p.o. q12h.
- Guinea pigs: 5 mg/kg i.m. q12h.
- Rats: 20 mg/kg i.m. q8–12h, 10–20 mg/kg p.o. q8h.
- Mice: 100 mg/kg s.c. q12h; 10–20 mg/kg p.o. q8h.

Birds:

- Raptors: 25–50 mg/kg p.o. q8h.
- Parrots: 50 mg/kg i.m. q24h; 200 mg/kg i.m. q24h – long-acting preparations.
- Passerines: 100 mg/kg p.o. q24h or 4–12 mg/l water for 7 days.
- Pigeons: 50 mg/kg p.o. q6h or 80 mg/kg i.m. q48h (long-acting preparations) or 130–400 mg/l water.

Reptiles: 6–10 mg/kg p.o., i.m., i.v. q24h.

NOTES

Oxytocin [16]

(Oxytocin S) POM-V

Formulations: Injectable: 10 IU/ml solution.

DOSES

Dogs:
- Obstetric indications: 0.1–0.5 IU/kg i.m., s.c. q30min for up to 3 doses.
- Milk let-down: 2–20 IU/dog i.m., s.c. once.

Cats:
- Obstetric indications: 0.1–0.5 IU/kg i.m., s.c. q30min for up to 2 doses.
- Milk let-down: 1–10 IU/cat i.m., s.c. once.

Small mammals:
- Ferrets: 0.2–3.0 IU/kg s.c., i.m.
- Rabbits: 0.1–3.0 IU/kg s.c., i.m.
- Rodents: 0.2–3 IU/kg s.c., i.m., i.v.
- Mice (milk let-down): 6.25 IU/kg s.c.

Birds: Do not use.

Reptiles: Egg retention: 2–10 IU/kg i.m. q90min; maximum of 3 doses. Better effect if calcium therapy used first.

NOTES

NOTES

NOTES

NOTES

Patellar luxations – grading[9]

Grade I

The patella can be manually luxated when the stifle is extended; however, when released it returns to the trochlea. Internal rotation of the tibia and displacement of the tibial tuberosity are minimal.

Grade II

The patella is frequently located medially with flexion of the stifle joint; however, it is easily reduced when the stifle is extended and the tibia externally rotated. The tibial tuberosity is displaced medially. Mild angular deformity of the femur and tibia may be present.

Grade III

The patella is permanently luxated. It may be reduced, but luxation recurs immediately. Angular and rotational deformities of the femur and tibia are common. The trochlea is usually shallow or flat.

Grade IV

The patella is permanently luxated and it is not possible manually to reposition it in the trochlea. Muscle contracture reduces the range of stifle extension. Angular and rotational deformity of the femur and tibia are generally marked and the tibial tuberosity is displaced 60–90 degrees medially. Concurrent external rotation of the distal tibia may result in reasonable alignment of the hock and hind paw. The trochlea is flat or convex.

NOTES

Percentage solutions conversion table[16]

The concentration of a solution may be expressed on the basis of weight per unit volume (w/v) or volume per unit volume (v/v).

% w/v = number of grams of a substance in 100 ml of a liquid

% v/v = number of ml of a substance in 100 ml of liquid

% Solution	g or ml/100 ml	mg/ml	Solution strength
100	100	1000	1:1
10	10	100	1:10
1	1	10	1:100
0.1	0.1	1	1:1000
0.01	0.01	0.1	1:10,000

Pimobendan[16]

(Cardisure, Vetmedin) POM-V

Formulations: Oral: 1.25 mg, 2.5 mg, 5 mg, 10 mg capsules.

DOSES

Dogs, Cats: 0.1–0.3 mg/kg p.o. q12h one hour before food.
A target dose of 0.25 mg/kg p.o. q12h is recommended in dogs.

Vetmedin (from datasheet)				
Dose rate	Patient bodyweight (kg)	Daily dosage (mg)	No. of tablets required, twice daily	
			1.25 mg	*5.0 mg*
Dogs				
0.2–0.6 mg/kg	<5	1.25	½	
	5–10	2.5	1	
	11–20	5		½
	21–40	10		1
	41–60	20		2
	>60	30		3

Polyuria/polydipsia (PU/PD) – diagnostic approach[10]

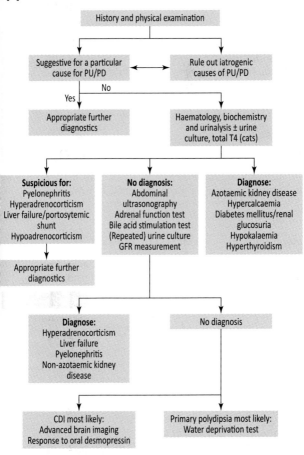

History and physical examination

Suggestive for a particular cause for PU/PD ⟷ Rule out iatrogenic causes of PU/PD

Yes / No

Appropriate further diagnostics

Haematology, biochemistry and urinalysis ± urine culture, total T4 (cats)

Suspicious for:
Pyelonephritis
Hyperadrenocorticism
Liver failure/portosytemic shunt
Hypoadrenocorticism

Appropriate further diagnostics

No diagnosis:
Abdominal ultrasonography
Adrenal function test
Bile acid stimulation test
(Repeated) urine culture
GFR measurement

Diagnose:
Azotaemic kidney disease
Hypercalcaemia
Diabetes mellitus/renal glucosuria
Hypokalaemia
Hyperthyroidism

Diagnose:
Hyperadrenocorticism
Liver failure
Pyelonephritis
Non-azotaemic kidney disease

No diagnosis

CDI most likely:
Advanced brain imaging
Response to oral desmopressin

Primary polydipsia most likely:
Water deprivation test

CDI = central diabetes insipidus; GFR = glomerular filtration rate

Potassium salts[16] (Potassium chloride, Potassium gluconate)

(Kaminox, Tumil-K) POM, AGM-GSL

Formulations:

- Injectable: 15% KCl solution (150 mg KCl/ml; 2 mmol/ml K^+ and Cl^-). Dilute with at least 25 times its own volume before i.v. administration.
- Oral: Tablets containing 2 mEq potassium gluconate; Powder (2 mEq per 1/4 teaspoon) (Tumil-K); Liquid 1 mEq/ml potassium gluconate formulated with a range of amino acids, B vitamins and iron (Kaminox). Note: 1 mmol/l =1 mEq/l.

DOSES

Dogs:

- Intravenous: Doses must be titrated for each patient; dilute concentrated solutions prior to use (normally to 20–60 mmol/l) Rate of i.v. infusion should not exceed 0.5 mmol/kg/h, especially when concentration in replacement fluid is >60 mmol/l. Use of fluid pumps is recommended.

Serum potassium	Amount to add to 250 ml 0.9% NaCl
<2 mmol/l	20 mmol
2–2.5 mmol/l	15 mmol
2.5–3 mmol/l	10 mmol
3–3.5 mmol/l	7 mmol
3.5–5.5 mmol/l	5 mmol (minimum daily need in anorectic patients)

- Oral: Replacement dose needs to be titrated to effect to maintain mid-range normal values in each individual patient. Starting doses are 2 mEq per 4.5 kg in food q12h or 2.2 mEq per 100 kcal required energy intake.

Cats:

- Intravenous: Doses as for dogs.
- Oral: Replacement dose needs to be titrated to effect to maintain mid-range normal values in each individual patient. Starting doses are 2.2 mEq per 4.5 kg in food q12h or 2–6 mEq/cat/day p.o. in divided doses q8–12h.

NOTES

Praziquantel [16]

(Bob Martin Spot-on Dewormer, Cazitel, Cestem, Dolpac, Droncit, Drontal cat, Drontal plus, Exitel, Milbemax, Plerion, Prazitel, Profender) POM-V, NFA-VPS, VPM-AVM, GSL

Formulations:

- Injectable: 56.8 mg/ml solution.
- Oral: 50 mg and 175 mg praziquantel with pyrantel and febantel tablets (Cazitel, Cestem, Drontal plus, Exitel, Prazitel); 10 mg, 50 mg and 125 mg praziquantel with oxantel and pyrantel tablets (Dolpac, Plerion); 20 mg, 30 mg praziquantel with pyrantel tablets (Drontal cat); 25 mg, 125 mg praziquantel with milbemycin tablets (Milbemax for dogs); 10 mg, 40 mg praziquantel with milbemycin tablets (Milbemycin for cats). Topical: 20 mg, 30 mg, 60 mg, 96 mg in spot-on pipette (Bob Martin Spot-on Dewormer, Droncit); 85.8 mg/ml praziquantel with emodepside in spot-on pipettes (Profendor).

DOSES

Dogs: 3.5–7.5 mg/kg i.m., s.c.; 5 mg/kg p.o.; 8 mg/kg spot-on.

Cats: 3.5–7.5 mg/kg i.m., s.c.; 5 mg/kg p.o.; 8 mg/kg spot-on.

Small mammals:
- Ferrets: 5–10 mg/kg p.o., s.c., i.m. repeated in 10–14 days.
- Rabbits: 5–10 mg/kg p.o., s.c., i.m. repeated in 10 days.
- Gerbils, Rats, Mice: 30 mg/kg p.o. q14d (for 3 treatments).

Birds:
- Pigeons: 10–20 mg/kg p.o. or 7.5 mg/kg s.c.
- Other birds: 10 mg/kg i.m., repeat after 7–10 days.

Reptiles: 5–8 mg/kg p.o., repeat after 2 weeks in most species.

Drontal (from datasheet)

Dose rate	Patient bodyweight (kg)	No. of tablets required
Dogs		
15 mg/kg bodyweight febantel, 14.4 mg/kg pyrantel and 5 mg/kg praziquantel	**Drontal Plus Flavour Tablets / Drontal Plus Flavour Bone Shaped Tablets**	
	3–5	½
	6–10	1
	11–15	1½
	16–20	2
	21–25	2½
	26–30	3
	31–35	3 ½
	36–40	4
	Drontal Plus XL Flavour Tablets	
	<17.5	½
	>17.5–35	1
	>35–52.5	1½
	>52.5–70	2
Cats		
57.5 mg/kg bodyweight pyrantel embonate and 5 mg/kg praziquantel	**Drontal Cat Tablets**	
	2 kg	½
	4 kg	1
	6 kg	1½
	8 kg	2
	Drontal Cat XL Film-coated Tablets	
	6	1

NOTES

Prednisolone [16]

(PLT, Prednicare, Prednidale, Prednisolone, Pred forte*) POM-V

Formulations:

- Ophthalmic: Prednisolone acetate 0.5%, 1% suspensions in 5 ml, 10 ml bottles (Pred forte).
- Topical: Prednisolone is a component of many topical dermatological, otic and ophthalmic preparations.
- Injectable: Prednisolone sodium succinate 10 mg/ml solution; 7.5 mg/ml suspension plus 2.5 mg/ml dexamethasone.
- Oral: 1 mg, 5 mg, 25 mg tablets. PLT is a compound preparation containing cinchophen.

DOSES

Dogs:

- Ophthalmic: Dosage frequency and duration of therapy is dependent upon type of lesion and response to therapy. Usually 1 drop in affected eye(s) q4–24h tapering in response to therapy.
- Allergy: 0.5–1.0 mg/kg p.o. q12h initially, tapering to lowest q48h dose.
- Anti-inflammatory: 0.5 mg/kg p.o. q12–24h; taper to 0.25–0.5 mg/kg q48h.
- Immunosuppression: 1.0–2.0 mg/kg p.o. q24h, tapering slowly to 0.5 mg/kg q48h (for many conditions this will take 6 months).
- Hypoadrenocorticism: 0.2–0.3 mg/kg with fludrocortisone. The use of prednisolone may be discontinued in most cases once the animal is stable.
- Lymphoma: see *BSAVA Small Animal Formulary*.

Cats:

- Ophthalmic, Allergy, Hypoadrenocorticism: Doses as for dogs.
- Anti-inflammatory: 0.5–1.0 mg/kg p.o. q12–24h; taper to 0.5 mg/kg q48h.
- Immunosuppression: 1.0–2.0 mg/kg p.o. q12–24h, tapering slowly to 0.5–1.0 mg/kg q48h (for many conditions this will take 6 months).
- Lymphoma: see *BSAVA Small Animal Formulary*.

Small mammals:

- Ferrets: lymphoma, anti-inflammatory: 1–2 mg/kg p.o. q24h (see *BSAVA Manual of Rodents and Ferrets* for specific protocols for lymphoma); postoperative management of adrenalectomy: 0.25–0.5 mg/kg p.o. q12h, taper to q48h.
- Rabbits: anti-inflammatory: 0.25–0.5 mg/kg p.o. q12h for 3 days, then q24h for 3 days, then q48h.
- Others: anti-inflammatory: 1.25–2.5 mg/kg p.o. q24h.

Birds: Pruritus: 1 mg/kg p.o. q12h, reduced to minimum effective dose as quickly as possible.

Reptiles:

- Analgesic, Anti-inflammatory: 2–5 mg/kg p.o. q 24–48h.
- Lymphoma: 40 mg/m^2 q48h with chlorambucil 2 mg/m^2 q24h q30d.

Premedication protocols – drug combinations used in dogs and cats[4]

Drug combination	
Drug 1	**Drug 2**
Acepromazine (0.03–0.05 mg/kg)	/ Methadone (0.2–0.5 mg/kg) / Morphine (0.2–0.5 mg/kg) / Hydromorphone (0.05–0.15 mg/kg) / Pethidine (meperidine) (4–5 mg/kg) / Buprenorphine (0.02 mg/kg) / Butorphanol (0.2–0.4 mg/kg)
Medetomidine (0.01–0.02 mg/kg) Or Dexmedetomidine (0.005–0.01 mg/kg) (use lower end of dose range in dogs >35 kg bodyweight to take account of metabolic size)	/ Buprenorphine (0.02 mg/kg) / Butorphanol (0.2–0.4 mg/kg) / Hydromorphone (0.1 mg/kg) / Morphine (0.1–0.2 mg/kg) / Methadone (0.1–0.2 mg/kg) / Midazolam (0.2–0.3 mg/kg) / Diazepam (0.2–0.3 mg/kg)
Midazolam (0.3–0.4 mg/kg)	/ Methadone (0.2–0.5 mg/kg) / Morphine (0.2–0.5 mg/kg) / Hydromorphone (0.05–0.15 mg/kg)
Midazolam (0.2–0.3 mg/kg)	/ Ketamine (5–10 mg/kg)
Zolazepam + tiletamine	Available as a proprietary mixture (Telazol or Zoletil) Dose range for premedication 3–6 mg/kg
Morphine (0.2–0.5 mg/kg) Methadone (0.2–0.5 mg/kg) Hydromorphone (0.05–0.1 mg/kg)	

Route of administration	Species	Patient selection
i.m. or i.v. i.m. i.m. or i.v. i.m. i.v., i.m., s.c.	Cat and dog Cat and dog Cat and dog Cat and dog Cat and dog	ASA 1–3 patients depending on assessment of cardiovascular function. Use lower dose of acepromazine in ASA 2–3 patients. Use lower dose range of drugs when given intravenously
i.m. or i.v. i.m. or i.v. i.m. or i.v. i.m. i.m. or i.v. Use lower doses i.v.	Cat and dog Cat and dog Cat and dog Cat and dog Cat and dog	ASA 1–2 patients. Cardiovascular function must be normal
i.m. or i.v. – use lower dose i.v.	Dog Dog	ASA 1–2 patients. Cardiovascular function must be normal. Useful for non-painful procedures such as diagnostic imaging
i.m. or i.v. i.m. i.v. or i.m.	Dog Dog Dog, rarely cat	ASA 3–5 Good cardiovascular stability
i.m. or i.v. – use lower dose i.v.	Cat	ASA 2–4. Avoid in patients with hypertrophic cardiomyopathy. Higher dose of ketamine will induce anaesthesia
i.m. or i.v. – use lower dose i.v.	Cat and dog	As above for midazolam/ketamine mixture. Recovery can be stormy in dogs
i.m. i.m. or i.v. i.m. or i.v.	Cat and dog Use lower end of dose range and intramuscular route in cats	ASA 4–5 Young animals

ASA = American Society of Anesthesiologists; *see* **ASA scale**.

see also **Acepromazine, Dexmedetomidine and Medetomidine**.

NOTES

NOTES

Prescribing cascade [16]

When no authorized veterinary medicinal product exists for a condition in a particular species, and in order to avoid unacceptable suffering, veterinary surgeons exercising their clinical judgement may prescribe for one or a small number of animals under their care other suitable medications in accordance with the following sequence:

1. A veterinary medicine authorized for use in another species, or for a different use in the same species ('off-label' use)
2. A medicine authorized in the UK for human use or a veterinary medicine from another country with an import certificate from the Veterinary Medicines Directorate (VMD)
3. A medicine to be made up at the time on a one-off basis by a veterinary surgeon or a properly authorized person.

Pruritus – diagnostic approach[7]

Dogs

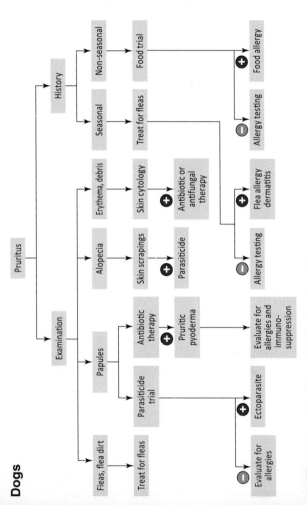

Cats

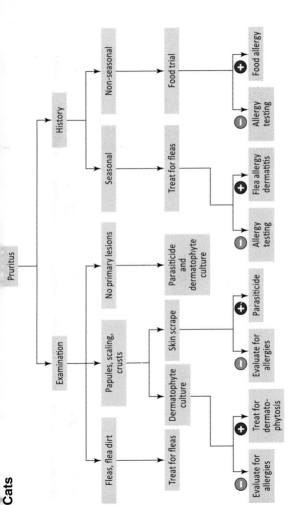

PUPD *see* Polyuria/polydipsia (PU/PD) – diagnostic approach

Pyoderma investigation[7]

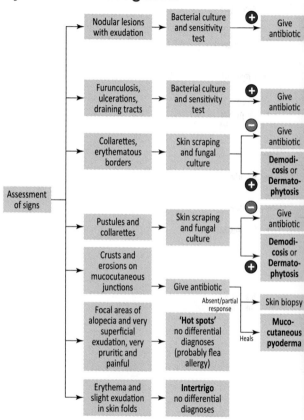

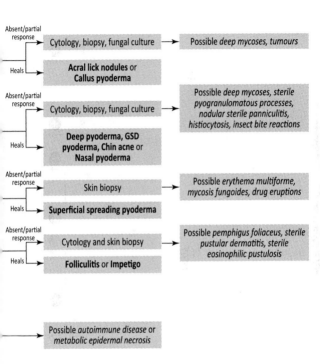

Absent/partial response → Cytology, biopsy, fungal culture → Possible *deep mycoses, tumours*

Heals → **Acral lick nodules** or **Callus pyoderma**

Absent/partial response → Cytology, biopsy, fungal culture → Possible *deep mycoses, sterile pyogranulomatous processes, nodular sterile panniculitis, histiocytosis, insect bite reactions*

Heals → **Deep pyoderma, GSD pyoderma, Chin acne** or **Nasal pyoderma**

Absent/partial response → Skin biopsy → Possible *erythema multiforme, mycosis fungoides, drug eruptions*

Heals → **Superficial spreading pyoderma**

Absent/partial response → Cytology and skin biopsy → Possible *pemphigus foliaceus, sterile pustular dermatitis, sterile eosinophilic pustulosis*

Heals → **Folliculitis** or **Impetigo**

→ Possible *autoimmune disease* or *metabolic epidermal necrosis*

GSD = German Shepherd Dog

Pyrantel [16]

(Cazitel, Cestem, Dolpac, Drontal cat, Drontal plus, Drontal puppy, Exitel, Plerion, Prazitel) POM-V

Formulations: Oral: Pyrantel with praziquantel and febantel (50 mg, 50 mg, 150 mg; 175 mg, 175 mg, 525 mg) tablets (Cazitel, Cestem, Drontal plus, Exitel, Prazitel); pyrantel with praziquantel and oxantel (10 mg, 10 mg, 40 mg; 25 mg, 25 mg, 100 mg; 50 mg, 50 mg, 200 mg; 125 mg, 125 mg, 500 mg) tablets (Dolpac, Plerion); 230 mg, 345 mg pyrantel embonate with praziquantel tablets (Drontal cat); 14.4 mg/ml pyrantel embonate with 15 mg/ml febantel suspension (Drontal puppy). Note: some formulations and doses give content of pyrantel (febantel, oxantel) in terms of pyrantel embonate/pamonate (50 mg pyrantel is equivalent to 144 mg pyrantel embonate/pamonate).

DOSES

Dogs: 5 mg/kg pyrantel + 15 mg/kg febantel or 20 mg/kg oxantel p.o., repeat as required.

Cats: 57.5 mg/kg pyrantel embonate.

Small mammals:
- Ferrets: 4.4 mg/kg (pyrantel embonate) p.o., repeat in 14 days.
- Rabbits: 5–10 mg/kg (pyrantel embonate) p.o., repeat in 14 days.
- Rodents: 50 mg/kg (pyrantel embonate) p.o., repeat as required.

NOTES

NOTES

NOTES

NOTES

Rabbit biological data [14]

Lifespan (years)	5–12 (can be greater in some individuals)
Average weight (kg)	1–10 (breed-dependent)
Heart rate (beats/min)	180–300
Respiratory rate (breaths/min)	30–60 (higher if stressed)
Blood volume (ml/kg)	Approximately 60
Rectal temperature (°C)	38.5–40.0
Dentition	2 [I2/1 C0/0 P3/2 M3/3]
Daily water intake (ml/kg)	50–150
Daily urine production (ml/kg)	10–35
Food intake per day (g/kg)	50
Sexual maturity	4–8 months (does earlier than bucks)
Oestrous cycle	Induced (reflex) ovulation; oestrus January–October
Length of gestation	28–32 days
Litter size	4–12
Birth weight	30–80 g
Weaning age	6 weeks

NOTES

Ranitidine[16]

(Ranitidine*, Zantac*) POM

Formulations:

- Injectable: 25 mg/ml solution.
- Oral: 75, 150, 300 mg tablets; 15 mg/ml syrup.

DOSES

Dogs: 2 mg/kg slow i.v., s.c., p.o. q8–12h.

Cats: 2 mg/kg/day constant i.v. infusion, 2.5 mg/kg i.v. slowly q12h, 3.5 mg/kg p.o. q12h.

Small mammals:

- Ferrets: 3.5 mg/kg p.o. q12h.
- Rabbits: 4–6 mg/kg p.o., s.c. q8–24h.
- Chinchillas, Guinea pigs: 5 mg/kg p.o. q12h as a prokinetic.

Rat biological data[14]

Lifespan (years)	2–3.5
Average weight (g) **Males:** **Females:**	270–500 225–325
Number of digits **Front:** **Rear:**	4 5
Heart rate (beats/min)	310–500
Respiratory rate (breaths/min)	70–150
Rectal temperature (°C)	~38
Dentition	2 [I1/1 C0/0 P0/0 M3/3] Only incisors open-rooted
Environmental temperature (°C)	21–24
Relative humidity (%)	45–55
Daily water intake	10 ml/100 g
Fluid therapy	100 ml/kg/24h
Diet	Omnivorous

Food intake per day per animal (g)	15–20
Coprophagy/Caecotrophy?	Yes
Oestrous type	Continuous polyoestrous
Post-partum oestrus?	Yes
Age at puberty (months)	1
Gestation length (days)	21–23
Oestrous cycle (days)	4–5
Oestrus duration (hours)	9–20
Litter size	6–13
Birth weight (g)	4–6
Altricial/Precocial	Altricial
Eyes open (days)	12–15
Age at weaning (days)	21
Number of pairs of teats	6
Minimum breeding age (months)	2
Ratio for breeding (M:F)	1:1–6 If polygamous remove female on day 16
Comments	They will eat the litter if disturbed in the first 2–3 days

NOTES

Respiratory distress algorithm [5]

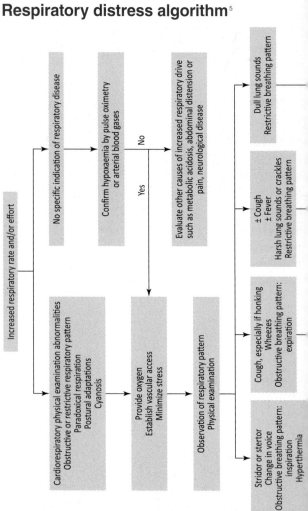

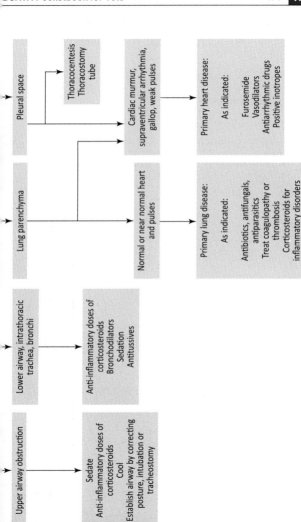

Resting energy requirement calculation[12]

RER (kcal) = 70 × bodyweight (kg) $^{0.75}$

or

RER (kcal) = 30 × bodyweight (kg) + 70

To convert kcal (Cal) to kilojoules (kJ) multiply by 4.185

NOTES

NOTES

NOTES

Schirmer tear test reference values[3]

Dogs	Mean reference value = 20 mm/min <10 mm/min raises suspicion of keratoconjunctivitis sicca (KCS) <5 mm/min diagnostic for KCS
Cats	Mean reference value = 17 mm/min <5 mm/min raises suspicion of KCS

NOTES

Sedation combinations [4]

For dogs and cats

Drug combination	
Drug 1	**Drug 2**
Medetomidine (0.02–0.04 mg/kg) Or Dexmedetomidine (0.01–0.02 mg/kg) (use lower end of dose range in dogs >35 kg bodyweight to take account of metabolic size)	/ Buprenorphine (0.02 mg/kg) / Butorphanol (0.2–0.4 mg/kg) / Hydromorphone (0.1 mg/kg)
	/ Midazolam (0.3 mg/kg) / Diazepam (0.3 mg/kg)
Acepromazine (0.03–0.05 mg/kg)	/ Methadone (0.2–0.5 mg/kg) / Morphine (0.2–0.5 mg/kg) / Pethidine (4–5 mg/kg) as above / Buprenorphine (0.02 mg/kg) / Butorphanol (0.2–0.4 mg/kg) / Hydromorphone (0.1–0.2 mg/kg)
Midazolam (0.4–0.5 mg/kg)	/ Methadone (0.2–0.5 mg/kg) / Morphine (0.2–0.5 mg/kg) / Hydromorphone (0.1–0.15 mg/kg)
Midazolam (0.2–0.3 mg/kg)	/ Ketamine (5–10 mg/kg)
Zolazepam + tiletamine	Available as a proprietary mixture (Telazol or Zoletil) Dose range for sedation/short duration general anaesthesia 9–13 mg/kg
Morphine (0.2–0.5 mg/kg) Methadone (0.2–0.5 mg/kg) Hydromorphone (0.1–0.2 mg/kg)	

Route of administration	Species notes	Sedation notes
i.m. or i.v. Use lower doses i.v.	Dogs and cats	Higher doses of medetomidine will provide more reliable and profound sedation. Expect animals to become recumbent. Useful for invasive painful procedures such as removal of grass seeds from the ear canal
i.m. or i.v. Use lower doses i.v.	Dogs	Higher doses of medetomidine will provide more reliable and profound sedation. Expect animals to become recumbent. Degree of analgesia is less than when medetomidine is combined with an opioid
i.v. or i.m. i.m. i.m. i.m. or i.v. i.m. or i.v. Use lower doses i.v.	Dogs: higher doses of opioids will provide greater sedation Cats: use low to mid dose range of opioids	Will provide light sedation in cats and dogs. Do not expect animals to become recumbent
i.m. or i.v. i.m. i.m. or i.v.	Dogs	Degree of sedation will depend on the health and temperament of the patient. May be able to carry out some invasive procedures if the animal is handled patiently and quietly
i.m. or i.v. – use lower doses i.v.	Cats	Expect profound sedation/light general anaesthesia
i.m. or i.v. – use lower doses i.v.	Dogs and cats	As above for midazolam/ ketamine mixture. Recovery can be stormy in dogs
i.m. i.m. or i.v. i.m. or i.v.	Dogs and cats Use lower end of dose range and intramuscular route in cats	Mild sedation only. Do not expect animal to become recumbent

For exotic pets

Ferrets:

- Ketamine (5–8 mg/kg i.m.) plus medetomidine (80–100 μg (micrograms)/kg) i.m.) or dexmedetomidine (30 μg (micrograms)/kg i.m.) to which can be added butorphanol (0.1–0.2 mg/kg i.m.) or buprenorphine (0.02 mg/kg i.m.).
- Ketamine (10–25 mg/kg i.m.) plus xylazine (2 mg/kg i.m.) to which can be added butorphanol (0.1–0.2 mg/kg i.m.) or buprenorphine (0.02 mg/kg i.m.).
- Ketamine (5–20 mg/kg i.m.) plus midazolam (0.25–0.5 mg/kg i.m.) or diazepam (0.25–0.5 mg/kg i.m.) will provide immobilization or, at the higher doses, a short period of anaesthesia.

Rabbits:

- Ketamine (15 mg/kg s.c.) plus medetomidine (250 μg (micrograms)/kg s.c.) to which can be added butorphanol (0.1–0.4 mg/kg s.c.).
- Ketamine (40–50 mg/kg i.m. or 200 mg/kg i.p.) plus xylazine (2–5 mg/kg i.m. or 10 mg/kg i.p.) or diazepam (1 mg/kg i.m. or 2.5 mg/kg i.p.).
- Fentanyl/fluanisone (0.3 ml/kg i.m. plus diazepam (1 mg/kg i.v., i.m. or 2.5–5.0 mg/kg i.p.) or midazolam (1.0–2.5 mg/kg i.v., i.m., i.p.).

Other small mammals:

- Medetomidine (50 μg (micrograms)/kg i.m.) or dexmedetomidine (25 μg (micrograms)/kg i.m.) plus, if needed, ketamine (2–4 mg/kg i.m.).
- Other combinations as for rabbits.

NB. Reduce doses if animal is debilitated.

Birds:

Injectable anaesthesia is best avoided unless in field situations (i.e. no gaseous anaesthesia available) or for the induction of large (e.g. swans/ratites), diving (e.g. ducks) or high-altitude birds. Even in these species, gaseous induction and maintenance (e.g. with ~rane/sevoflurane) would still be the normal recommendation ~ver possible. Sedation and premedicants are rarely used, as ~ndling will add to the general stress of the situation.

On occasions, diazepam (0.2–0.5 mg/kg i.m.) or midazolam (0.1–0.5 mg/kg i.m.) may be used; alternatively, either drug may be used at 0.05–0.15 mg/kg i.v. Parasympatholytic agents (such as atropine) are rarely used as their effect is to make respiratory secretions more viscous, thus increasing the risk of tube blockage.

- Propofol (10 mg i.v. by slow infusion to effect: supplemental doses up to 3 mg/kg).
- Alfaxalone (2–4 mg/kg i.v.) is an alternative to propofol for the induction of anaesthesia in large birds or those with a dive response.
- Ketamine/diazepam combinations can be used for induction and muscle relaxation. Ketamine (30–40 mg/kg) plus diazepam (1.0–1.5 mg/kg) are given slowly i.v. to effect. May also be given i.m. but this produces different effects in different species and specific literature or specialist advice should be consulted.
- Raptors: ketamine (2–5 mg/kg i.m.) plus medetomidine (25–100 µg (micrograms)/kg) (lower dose rate i.v.; higher rate i.m.). This combination can be reversed with atipamezole at 65 µg (micrograms)/kg i.m. Ketamine should be avoided in vultures.

Reptiles:
- Ketamine (20–60 mg/kg i.m. in chelonians; 25–60 mg/kg i.m. in lizards; 20–80 mg/kg i.m. in snakes). NB. Use lower end of dosage for sedation in all species. Recovery may be prolonged even with low dosages in debilitated, particularly renally compromised, patients. For such patients butorphanol (0.4 mg/kg i.m.) plus midazolam (2 mg/kg i.m.) may be safer.
- Ketamine (5–10 mg/kg i.m.) plus medetomidine (100–200 µg (micrograms)/kg) (deep sedation to light anaesthesia); may reverse medetomidine with atipamezole at 5 times the medetomidine dose (i.e. 0.5–1.0 mg/kg atipamezole).
- Ketamine (10–30 mg/kg i.m.) plus butorphanol (0.5–1 mg/kg i.m.) has also been recommended for deep sedation.
- Chelonians, snakes: sedation to light anaesthesia: ketamine (20–60 mg/kg i.m.) plus midazolam (1–2 mg/kg i.m.) or diazepam (chelonians: 0.2–1 mg/kg i.m.; snakes: 0.2–0.8 mg/kg i.m.).

- Alfaxalone (15 mg/kg i.m. or, preferably, 5–9 mg/kg i.v.) provides deep sedation/anaesthesia in chelonians (preferable to perform intermittent positive pressure ventilation with 100% oxygen after administration to prevent hypoxia).
- Midazolam (0.5–2 mg/kg i.m.) provides sedation for imaging and non-noxious procedures.
- Propofol (5–10 mg/kg i.v. or intraosseously) will give 10–15 minutes of sedation/light anaesthesia (preferable to perform intermittent positive pressure ventilation with 100% oxygen after administration to prevent hypoxia). May also be given intracoelomically to small chelonians.

See also Acepromazine, Dexmedetomidine, Diazepam, Ketamine **and** Medetomidine

NOTES

Selamectin [16]

(Stronghold) POM-V

Formulations: Topical: Spot-on pipettes of various sizes containing 6% or 12% selamectin.

DOSES

Dogs: Minimum dose recommendation 6 mg/kg. For effective treatment of sarcoptic mange apply product on three occasions at 2-week intervals.

Cats: Minimum dose recommendation 6 mg/kg as required.

Small mammals: Ferrets, Rabbits, Rodents: 6 mg/kg monthly.

Skunk biological data [14]

Lifespan (years)	8–10
Length (cm)	Head and body: 20–28 Tail: 28–43.5 (often carried over the back)
Bodyweight (kg)	0.75–4.0 Note: very fat skunks are frequently seen in practice
Body temperature (°C)	37.0–38.9
Heart rate (beats/min)	140–190
Respiratory rate (breaths/min)	35–40 (will pant when excited or hot)
Breeding season	February/March to May/June
Gestation period (days)	62–66
Average litter size	6
Weight at birth (g)	14
Lactation period	Up to 6 weeks
Weaning age	8 weeks

S-Methoprene *see* Methoprene

NOTES

Status epilepticus – clinical approach[11]

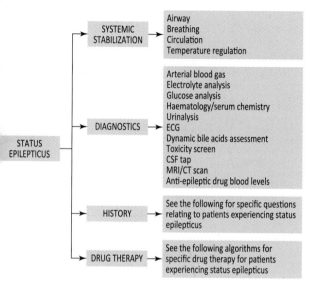

STATUS EPILEPTICUS	SYSTEMIC STABILIZATION	Airway Breathing Circulation Temperature regulation
	DIAGNOSTICS	Arterial blood gas Electrolyte analysis Glucose analysis Haematology/serum chemistry Urinalysis ECG Dynamic bile acids assessment Toxicity screen CSF tap MRI/CT scan Anti-epileptic drug blood levels
	HISTORY	See the following for specific questions relating to patients experiencing status epilepticus
	DRUG THERAPY	See the following algorithms for specific drug therapy for patients experiencing status epilepticus

approach to systemic stabilization and management of the status
epilepticus patient.

1. When did the episode start?
2. Is there a pre-existing seizure disorder?
3. Has the patient had status epilepticus or cluster seizure events before?
4. Have there been any systemic health problems within the last 4 months?
5. Has there been any change in the patient's personality or behaviour within the last 4 months?
6. Is the patient on medications including anticonvulsant therapy?
7. Which anticonvulsants are being given; what is the dose; when was the last dose?
8. How long has the patient been on anticonvulsants?
9. Have any recent serum anticonvulsant levels been performed?
10. Is there any recent trauma, travel history or toxin exposure?
11. Has the patient eaten a meal within the last few hours?

Important questions to ask about the patient in status epilepticus.

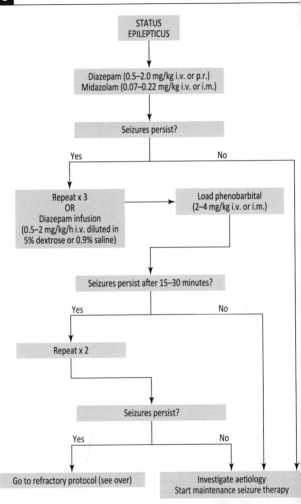

Approach to the initial pharmacological management of the status epilepticus patient.

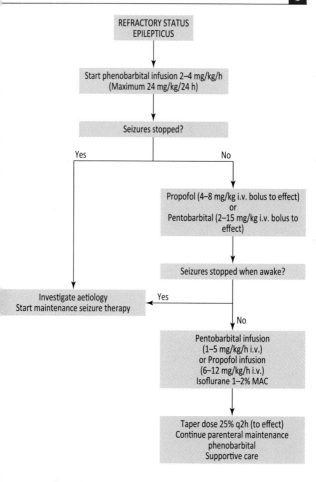

Approach to the pharmacological management of the refractory status epilepticus patient.

MAC = minimum alveolar concentration.

NOTES

NOTES

NOTES

Tepoxalin [16]

(Zubrin) POM-V

Formulations: Oral: 50 mg, 100 mg, 200 mg tablets.

DOSES

Dogs: 10 mg/kg p.o. q24h with food.

Cats: No published data. Do not use.

Thyroxine *see* Levothyroxine

Tibial compression test [3]

Indications/Use

- To diagnose partial or complete rupture of the cranial cruciate ligament (CCL)
- Note: not all dogs with CCL disease have femorotibial instability that can be detected by this test
- Often used in association with the cranial draw test

Patient preparation and positioning

- Can be performed in the conscious animal. However, if the patient is tense (due to pain or temperament) or if the CCL is only partially torn, sedation or general anaesthesia is required.
- A conscious patient should be restrained in a standing position on three legs, with the affected limb held off the ground.
- Sedated or anaesthetized patients may be positioned in lateral recumbency, with the affected limb uppermost.

Technique

1. Grasp and maintain the distal femur in a fixed position with one hand, placing the thumb over the lateral fabella and the index finger lightly on the tibial crest.
2. Use the other hand to grasp the metatarsal region.
3. Maintain the stifle joint in slight flexion, while slowly flexing the hock.

Results

■ Cranial displacement of the tibial crest relative to the femur is suggestive of CCL injury.

See also Cranial draw test

NOTES

Toxicological emergencies – initial management[8]

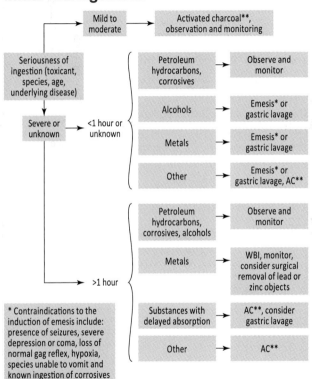

* Contraindications to the induction of emesis include: presence of seizures, severe depression or coma, loss of normal gag reflex, hypoxia, species unable to vomit and known ingestion of corrosives (acids or alkalis) or volatile petroleum hydrocarbons

** Single or multiple doses depending on toxicant ingested

AC = Activated charcoal; WBI = Whole bowel irrigation

Tramadol [16]

(Tramadol ER*, Ultracet*, Ultram*, Zamadol*) POM

Formulations:

- Oral: 50 mg tablets; 100 mg, 200 mg, 300 mg extended release tablets; 5 mg/ml oral liquid (only available by importation into the UK).
- Injectable: 50 mg/ml solution (only available by importation into the UK).

DOSES

Dogs: 2–5 mg/kg p.o. q8h, 2 mg/kg i.v.

Cats: 2–4 mg/kg p.o. q8h, 1–2 mg/kg i.v., s.c.

Small mammals: Rats: 10–20 mg/kg p.o., s.c.

Birds: 5 mg/kg p.o. q12h (bald eagles).

Tremors – diagnostic approach [11]

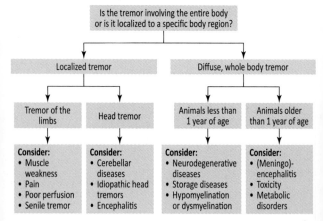

Trilostane [16]

(Vetoryl) POM-V

Formulations: Oral: 10 mg, 30 mg, 60 mg, 120 mg capsules.

DOSES

Dogs: 3–5 mg/kg p.o. q24h. Start at the low end of the range and increase gradually. Twice-daily dosing may be needed in some cases when clinical signs persist despite suppression of the cortisol response to ACTH stimulation. The total daily dose should be increased but not as much as doubled when switching from once to twice daily dosing.

Cats: 30 mg/cat p.o. q24h, adjusting dose according to clinical signs and post-treatment ACTH stimulation tests. Very few cats have been treated with trilostane.

NOTES

NOTES

NOTES

NOTES

Urine specific gravity[6]

Increased (>1.030 in dog, >1.035 in cat)

- Hypovolaemia
- Marked increase in glucose or protein content

Decreased (1.015–1.030 in dog, 1.015–1.035 in cat)

- Early renal failure
- Diabetes mellitus
- Hyperadrenocorticism
- May be normal (dog)

Isosthenuria (1.007–1.015) or Hyposthenuria (<1.007)

- Renal failure (I, H)
- Hyperadrenocorticism (I, H)
- Steroid therapy (I, H)
- Hypercalcaemia (I, H)
- Pyometra (I, H)
- Pyelonephritis (I, H)
- Renal medullary washout (e.g. post-obstruction) (I, H)
- Hyperthyroidism (I, rarely H)
- Psychogenic polydipsia (I, H)
- Fluid therapy (I, H)
- Liver disease (I, H)
- Partial central diabetes insipidus (I, H)
- Central or nephrogenic diabetes insipidus (usually H)

NOTES

NOTES

NOTES

NOTES

Weight loss strategy[12]

1. Determine the target weight of the animal (see *BSAVA Manual of Canine and Feline Rehabilitation, Supportive and Palliative Care: Case Studies in Patient Management*).

2. Calculate required energy intake.

Dogs

Calculate maintenance energy requirement (MER) at target bodyweight (TBW)

     e.g. $MER (kcal) = 132 \times TBW (kg)^{0.73}$

Decide upon the degree of caloric restriction for the animal, based upon sex and neuter status

e.g.	Entire male:	60% of MER
	Entire female:	55% of MER
	Neutered male:	55% of MER
	Neutered female:	50% of MER

Cats

Estimated starting energy intake (kcal) for weight loss is usually 35–40 x TBW (kg).

If necessary, adjust the degree of restriction based upon individual circumstances:

Consider additional restriction if:
- Reduced activity level (e.g. concurrent orthopaedic disease; owner lifestyle allows limited time for initiating play activity)

Consider a lower degree of restriction if:
- Very active dog
- Owner desires a more gradual weight loss programme (e.g. to minimize the impact of possible begging activity)

3. Take account of owners' wishes to feed 'treats'

4. Calculate the equivalent amount of food for the desired energy intake (in grams for dried food; in sachets or tins for wet food)

5. Decide upon the feeding strategy:

e.g.   Number of meals

Use of a feeding toy

Use of a proportion of the food as treats

6. Switch to the new diet gradually, over a few days if necessary.

NOTES

NOTES

NOTES

NOTES

NOTES

NOTES

References

1. *BSAVA/VPIS Guide to Common Canine and Feline Poisons* (2012)

2. *BSAVA* **companion**: How to pick your way through the jungle of ectoparasite treatments for dogs and cats (January 2012), by P. Lau-Gillard

3. *BSAVA Guide to Procedures in Small Animal Practice* (2010), ed. N. Bexfield and K. Lee

4. *BSAVA Manual of Canine & Feline Anaesthesia and Analgesia, 2nd edn* (2007), ed. C. Seymour and T. Duke-Novakovski

5. *BSAVA Manual of Canine & Feline Cardiorespiratory Medicine, 2nd edn* (2010), ed. V. Luis Fuentes, L.R. Johnson and S. Dennis

6. *BSAVA Manual of Canine & Feline Clinical Pathology, 2nd edn* (2005), ed. E. Villiers and L. Blackwood

7. *BSAVA Manual of Canine & Feline Dermatology, 3rd edn* (2012), ed. H. Jackson and R. Marsella

8. *BSAVA Manual of Canine & Feline Emergency and Critical Care, 2nd edn* (2007), ed. L. King and A. Boag

9. *BSAVA Manual of Canine & Feline Musculoskeletal Disorders* (2006), ed. J.E.F. Houlton, J.L. Cook, J.F. Innes and S.J. Langley-Hobbs

10. *BSAVA Manual of Canine & Feline Nephrology and Urology, 2nd edn* (2007), ed. J. Elliott and G.F. Grauer

11. *BSAVA Manual of Canine & Feline Neurology, 3rd edn* (2004), ed. Simon Platt and Natasha Olby

12. *BSAVA Manual of Canine & Feline Rehabilitation, Supportive and Palliative Care: Case Studies in Patient Management* (2010) ed. S. Lindley and P. Watson

13. *BSAVA Manual of Canine & Feline Thoracic Imaging* (2008), ed. T. Schwarz and V. Johnson

14. *BSAVA Manual of Exotic Pets, 5th edn* (2010), ed. A. Meredith and C. Johnson-Delaney

15. *BSAVA Manual of Small Animal Practice Management and Development* (2012), ed. C. Clarke and M. Chapman

16. *BSAVA Small Animal Formulary, 7th edn* (2011), editor-in-chief, I. Ramsey

17. *BSAVA Manual of Canine & Feline Ophthalmology, 2nd edn* (2002), ed. S. Petersen-Jones and S. Crispin

18. *Veterinary Ophthalmology, 4th edn (2007)*, ed. K.N. Gelatt. Lippincott, Williams and Wilkins, Philadelphia

19. *BSAVA* **companion**: How to approach the hypertensive patient (March 2012), by R.E. Jepson

Index of trade names

---

* Products that are not authorized for veterinary use by the Veterinary Medicines Directorate